SURGERY - PROCEDURES, COMPLICATIONS, AND RESULTS

SURGERY OF THE ORBITAL CAVITY

"NO-MAN'S-LAND"

SURGERY - PROCEDURES, COMPLICATIONS, AND RESULTS

Additional books in this series can be found on Nova's website
under the Series tab.

Additional e-books in this series can be found on Nova's website
under the e-book tab.

SURGERY - PROCEDURES, COMPLICATIONS, AND RESULTS

SURGERY OF THE ORBITAL CAVITY

"NO-MAN'S-LAND"

RADMILO RONCEVIC

NOVA BIOMEDICAL

New York

NOTICE TO THE READER

The Publisher has taken reasonable care in the preparation of this book, but makes no expressed or implied warranty of any kind and assumes no responsibility for any errors or omissions. No liability is assumed for incidental or consequential damages in connection with or arising out of information contained in this book. The Publisher shall not be liable for any special, consequential, or exemplary damages resulting, in whole or in part, from the readers' use of, or reliance upon, this material. Any parts of this book based on government reports are so indicated and copyright is claimed for those parts to the extent applicable to compilations of such works.

Independent verification should be sought for any data, advice or recommendations contained in this book. In addition, no responsibility is assumed by the publisher for any injury and/or damage to persons or property arising from any methods, products, instructions, ideas or otherwise contained in this publication.

This publication is designed to provide accurate and authoritative information with regard to the subject matter covered herein. It is sold with the clear understanding that the Publisher is not engaged in rendering legal or any other professional services. If legal or any other expert assistance is required, the services of a competent person should be sought. FROM A DECLARATION OF PARTICIPANTS JOINTLY ADOPTED BY A COMMITTEE OF THE AMERICAN BAR ASSOCIATION AND A COMMITTEE OF PUBLISHERS.

Additional color graphics may be available in the e-book version of this book.

Library of Congress Cataloging-in-Publication Data

ISBN: 978-1-63482-271-8
Library of Congress Control Number: 2015959371

Published by Nova Science Publishers, Inc. † New York

To my dear sisters Ikonija, Nada and Nevenka

Contents

Preface

Seen from the aspect of surgical interventions and surgery per se, the orbital cavity is still a "no-man's-land." None of the surgical disciplines completely encompasses the entire orbital spectrum, namely - orbital injuries, tumors and similar diseases, dysthyroid ophthalmopathy, congenital and acquired anomalies and deformities including lacrimal apparatus surgery.

Orbital surgery is customarily performed by specialists in ophthalmological surgery, neurosurgery, plastic and maxillofacial surgery, as well as specialists in otorhinolaringology. Surgery procedures are performed by using diverse surgical techniques and philosophy without a uniformed doctrine. Nowadays, specialists in craniofacial surgery successfully perform majority of complex orbital surgeries, with the exception of eyeball procedures, which exclusively fall within the scope of competence of a surgeon-ophthalmologist.

It is quite logical that orbital surgery belongs to craniofacial surgery, since the orbit is located in the center of the craniofacial region. In order to successfully perform a more complicated surgical procedure in the orbit, one must be familiar with the surrounding areas.

Exceptional knowledge of the orbital anatomy and the anatomy of its surrounding areas, is the first step in performing successful orbital surgery. As such, sufficient space in this book has been given to the anatomy of the orbit and the accessory visial structures. Irrespective of the fact that such information can be found in various textbooks of anatomy, I felt it was critical to include a comprehensive picture, in order to provide a complete understanding of the subject. In the chapter entitled "Anatomy of the Orbital Cavity" I mainly utilized the Jovanovic book, *Eye Cavity and the Visual Organ*, Scientific book, Belgrade, 1989. Certain details of importance to orbital surgery are stressed here, whereas these are not mentioned either in ordinary anatomy books or no major importance has been dedicated to them. Accompanying the text are sketches which have are based on Sinelnikov R. D., Sinelnikov JA. R., Sinelnikov A. JA.: Atlas of human anatomy, Novaja volna, Moscow, 2007-2010.

The chapters entitled "Treatment of Orbital Fractures," "Surgery of the Orbital Tumors" and "Surgical Treatment of Dysthyroid Ophthalmopathy" were written based on my own personal experience, my works published in peer reviewed journals, and the experiences of the most distinguished world experts in craniofacial surgery.

Since lacrimal surgery is a discipline of ophthalmology and not craniofacial surgery, I did not have the opportunity to be frequently engaged in this kind of surgery. Therefore, the chapter "Lacrimal Apparatus Surgery" was written based on experiences of the experts predominantly practicing this surgery.

Congenital craniofacial malformations with orbital malformations are not rarities. However, because these malformations require thorough, complex and risky surgical procedures, to which the patients or their parents often do not consent, the number of surgical procedures is limited in this area. The chapter titled "Surgery of Congenital Orbital Malformations" has been written based on major experiences of experts almost exclusively practicing this kind of surgery, along with my own personal experience.

All of the patients shown throughout this book are patients that I have personally operated on. The given results have been presented at international congresses, and have been published in peer reviewed journals.

Again, the intention of this book is to provide a comprehensive insight into orbital surgery, (excluding eyeball surgery), and to enable our young colleagues starting this difficult path to quickly overcome any hurdles which may pop up. Whilst the orbit represents the center of craniofacial region, this book can be of assistance to all specialists concentrated on this region. Particularly as a reference book about the possibilities and purposefulness of certain surgical procedures in the orbital region and its surrounding area to post-graduates in the field of ophthalmology, plastic and maxillofacial surgery, neurosurgery and otorhinolaryngology.

This book was made possible by my patients, associates and colleagues. I extend my deepest and most sincere gratitude to all of my patients for their confidence, cooperation, and patience, and to the entire team of the Clinic for Burns, Plastic and Reconstructive Surgery of the Clinical Centre of Serbia, where I have performed most of my surgeries.

I also wish to thank in advance all those who will give constructive reviews and comments of this book, and suggestions for modifications and additions to the next edition.

Radmilo P. Rončević, MD, DMD, PhD

Chapter 1

Anatomy of the Orbital Cavity

Surgery of the orbit can never be mastered, nor can it be skillfully performed, without an exceptional knowledge of orbital anatomy and its content (Figures 1-10).

The eye cavity - *orbit* (Figures 1, 2) is a paired bony structure, occupying 30 cm3 in volume, which lies bilaterally above the corresponding maxillary sinus, and below the anterior cranial cavity. The orbit has the shape of a four-sided pyramid with rounded angles, with the base positioned frontward, and the top turned backwards. The orbital axis, which goes from its apex to the base, is about 45 mm long and it is directed obliquely frontward, laterally, and slightly downwards. The axis of the right and the left orbit intersect forming a sharp angle turned to the front from 40 to 45 degrees. The base width is about 40 mm, and the height is 35 mm (1-5).

1.1. Orbital Base or Aperture (Aditus Orbitae)

The orbit base is directed frontward, laterally and downwards to form the orbital entrance. It is rectangular and has four margins: superior, inferior, lateral and medial.

The superior margin of the orbital aperture consists of the supraorbital margin *(margo supraorbitalis)* of the frontal bone. This margin is concave downwards and protruded frontward. The superior margin is sharp and protruded in the lateral half, and rounded in the medial one. This is where the supraorbital notch *(incisura supraorbitalis)* is located. This notch is closed from the floor by connective tissue, or a short bony bridge often turning it into a bony supraorital foramen *(foramen supraorbitalis).* The supraorbital artery and the lateral branch of the supraorbital nerve go through the supraorbital incisure i.e., opening. A few millimeters medially from the supraorbital incisure there is a considerably less distinct frontal notch *(incisura frontalis),* which, in extreme cases is turned into a frontal foramen *(foramen frontale).* The supratrochlear artery, and the medial branch of the supraorbital nerve pass through the frontal incisure or opening. A few millimeters above the medial half of the superior margin of the entrance into the orbit there is an arched protrusion – supraciliary arch *(arcus superciliaris),* which is more distinct in adult men than in women and children. The inferior margin of the orbital entrance consists of the infraorbital margin *(margo infraorbitalis)* of the maxilla, and partly of the anterior margin of the zygomatic bone. At 6 to 8 mm below the inferior margin of the orbital entrance there is the infraorbital foramen *(foramen infraorbitalis),* through which the infraorbital canal *(canalis infraorbitalis)* opens at the anterior part of the body of the maxilla. The infraorbtial artery and nerve (*a. et n. infraorbitalis)* go through the infraorbital canal and the opening. The lateral margin of the orbital entrance is thick and rounded and it consists of the anterior margin of the zygomatic bone. The medial margin of the orbital entrance is not clearly distinct in the larger, upper area. In the lower part, the anterior lacrimal crest *(crista lacrimalis anterior)* is well developed at the frontal process of the maxilla.

1.2. Orbital Walls

The orbit has four walls: superior, inferior, lateral and medial (Figures 1, 2). The superior wall *(paries superior),* or the orbital roof, is triangular and concave, particularly in the anterior part and it consists of: frontward – the lower side of the pars orbitalis of the frontal bone, and backwards – lesser wings of the sphenoid bone. In the anterolateral corner of the orbital superior wall there is the fossa of the lacrimal gland *(fossa glandulae lacrimalis),* in which the larger, orbital part of the gland is located. In the anteromedial corner of the superior orbital wall, around 5 mm behind the superior margin of the orbital aperture, there is a very shallow trochlear fovea *(fovea trochlearis),* in which the connective-cartilage trochlea of the superior oblique muscle is adjoined.

The inferior wall *(paries inferior)* or the orbital floor, runs obliquely downwards, frontward and laterally; it is thin and separates the orbit from the maxillary sinus cavity. The inferior wall is formed by three bones: the orbital side of the body of the maxilla, the orbital side of the zygomatic bone and the process of palatal bone, in the posterior medial corner of the orbit. In the anterior, bulbar part, the orbital floor is more or less concave, while the retrobulbar part is slightly convex. In the posterolateral part of the inferior wall of the orbit there is infraorbital groove (*sulcus infraorbitalis*), 3-4 mm wide, directed frontward and containing the infraorbital artery and the nerve. The infraorbital groove is bridged over by a thin periost of the orbit (periorbit) turning it into a bony-connective canal. The infraorbital groove, after a short path on the upper side of the body of the maxilla bends obliquely downwards and medially and enters the infraorbital canal *(canalis infraorbitalis),* that ends in the infraorbital opening at the anterior part of the body of the maxilla. In most cases the infraorbital canal is about 12 to 14 mm long and has four walls: superior, inferior, lateral and medial. The superior wall of the canal is occasionally very thin and separates the canal from the orbital floor.

The lateral wall *(paries lateralis*) is the thickest and the firmest orbital wall and it is formed by three bones: at the back – the orbital side of the grater wing of the sphenoid bone, at the front – the orbital side of the zygomatic bone, and at the front and upwards – the zygomatic process of the frontal bone. At the orbital side of the zygomatic bone, directly in front of the anterior end of the inferior orbital fissure and slightly above, there is a small round zygomaticoorbital opening *(foramen zygomaticoorbitalis).* Through this opening zygomatic nerve – the side branch of the maxillary nerve enters the zygomatic canal.

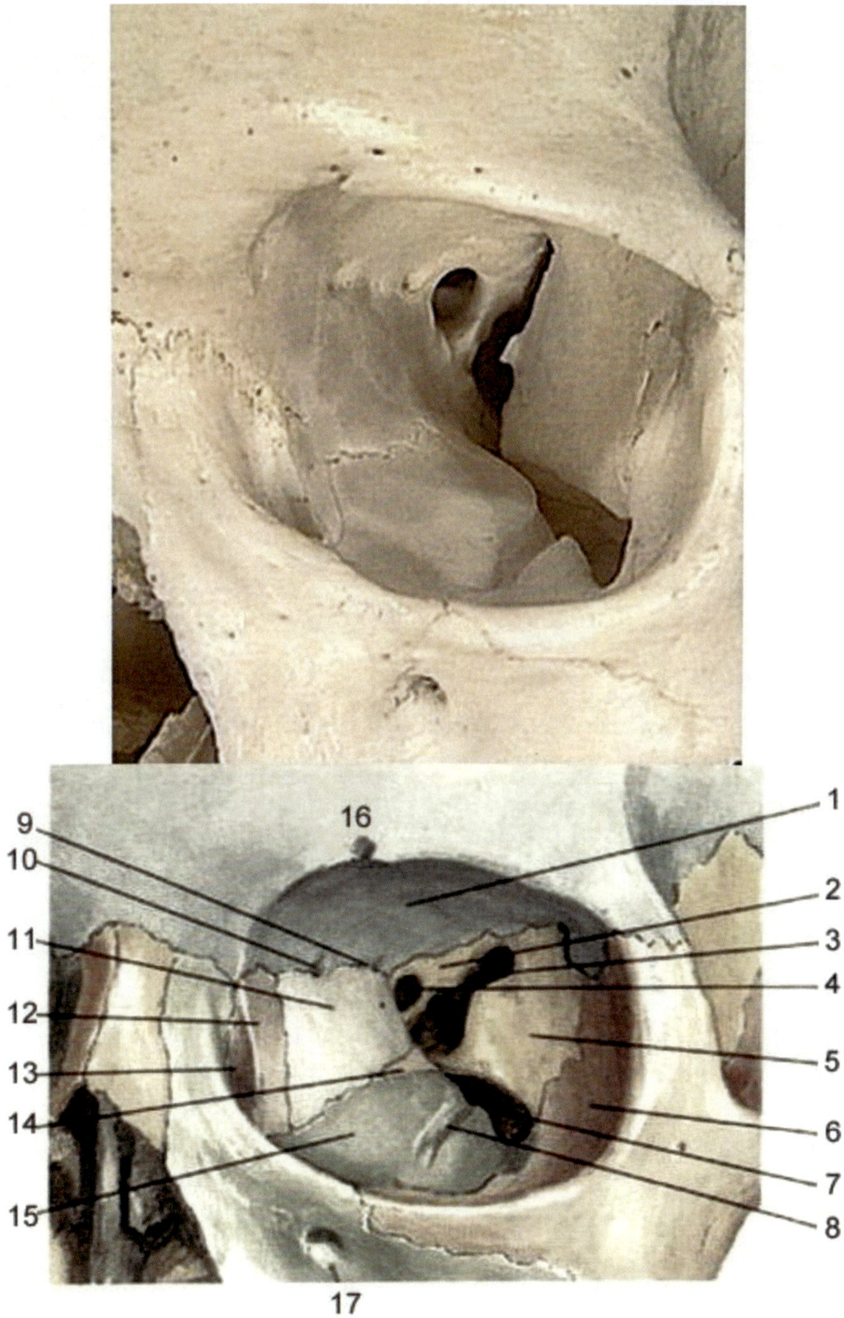

Figure 1. Bone structures of the orbit. 1 – Frontal bone, 2 – Lesser wing of sphenoid bone, 3 – Superior orbital fissure, 4 – Optic canal, 5 – Greater wing of sphenoid bone, 6 – Zygomatic bone, 7 – Inferior orbital fissure, 8 – Infraorbital sulcus, 9 – Posterior ethmoid foramen, 10 – Anterior ethmoid foramen, 11 – Orbital plate of the ethmoid bone, 12 – Lacrimal bone, 13 – Lacrimal fossa, 14 – Orbital process of the palatine bone, 15 – Maxilla, 16 – Supraorbital foramen 17 – Infraorbital foramen.

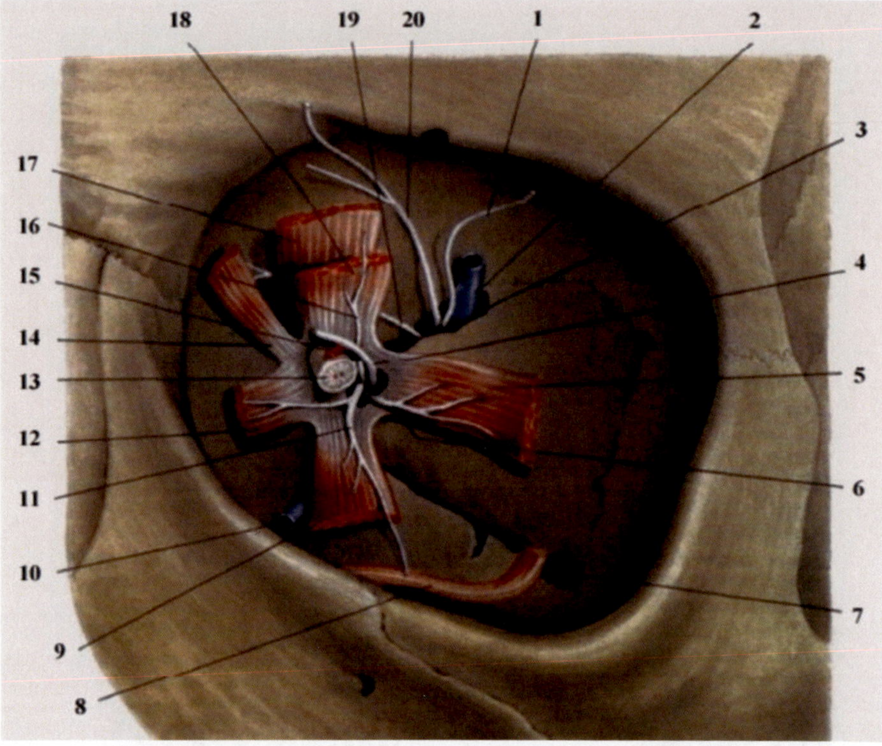

Figure 2. Apex of the orbit. 1 – Lacrimal nerve, 2 – Superior ophthalmic vein, 3 – Superior orbital fissure, 4 – Nasociliary nerve, 5 – Lateral rectus muscle, 6 – Abducens nerve, 7 – Inferior orbital fissure, 8 – Inferior oblique muscle, 9 – Inferior rectrus muscle, 10 – Inferior ophthalmic vein, 11 - Inferior division of oculomotor nerve, 12 – Medial rectus muscle, 13 – Optic nerve, 14 – Superior oblique muscle, 15 – Ophthalmic artery, 16 – Superior division of oculomotor nerve, 17 - Levator palpebrae superioris muscle, 18 – Superior rectus muscle, 19 – Trochlear nerve, 20 – Frontal nerve (Sketch is made on the base Sinelnikov R.D., Sinelnikov JA. R., Sinelnikov A. JA.: Atlas of human anatomy, Novaja volna, Moscow, 2007-2010).

The medial wall *(paries medialis)* is very thin and approximately rectangular, and it separates the eye cavity from the nasal cavity. This wall is formed by four bones: the frontal process (*processus frontalis)* of the maxilla, the lacrimal bone *(os lacrimale),* the orbital lamina *(lamina orbitalis)* of the ethmoid labyrinth and the anterior part of the lateral side of the sphenoid bone body. The three posterior quarters of the medial wall of the orbit are smooth and flat, and the anterior quarter makes the lacrimal fosa. The lacrimal fossa *(fossa sacci lacrimalis)* represents the bearing of the lacrimal sac. It is a vertical cavity 12-14 mm high and 3-4 mm wide. Anteriorly, the cavity is limited by the vertical anterior lacrimal crest *(crista lacrimalis anterior)* which is located on the frontal process of the maxilla, and posteriorly, by the posterior lacriml crest *(crista lacrimalis posterior)* which is at the lateral side of the lacrimal bone. The lacrimal fossa is formed by mutual connection of two vertical bony lacrimal grooves, the anterior, which belongs to the frontal process of the maxilla, and the posterior one, which belongs to the lacrimal bone. Both grooves are connected along a vertical lacrimomaxillary suture *(sutura lacrimomaxillaris),* which is visible at the floor of the lacrimal fossa. In the lower end the lacrimal fossa becomes deeper and it extends downwards into the bony naso-lacrimal canal *(canalis nasolacrimalis),* which opens into the nasal cavity immediately below the valut of inferior nasal meatus.

1.3. Orbital Corners

The orbit has four corners (Figures 1, 2, 3): superior lateral, superior medial, inferior lateral and inferior medial. Apart from the suture between the bones, there are openings and cracks in the orbital corners that connect the orbit with the surrounding regions.

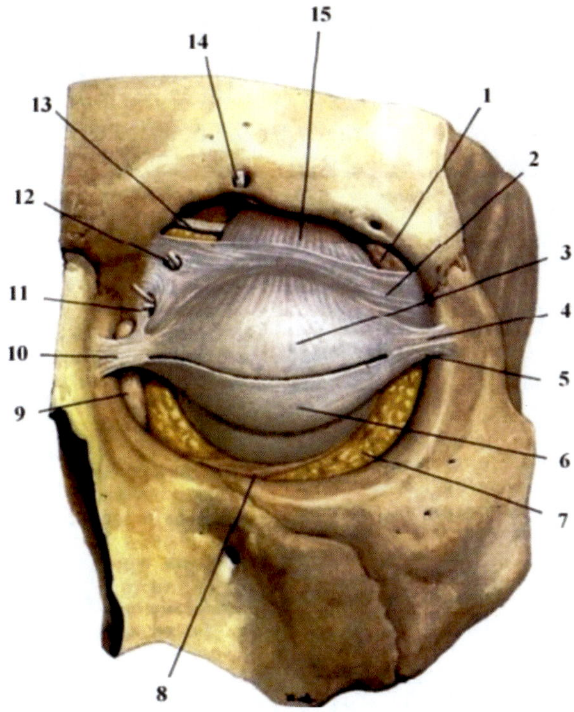

Figure 3. Anterior part of the orbit. 1 – Lacrimal gland (palpebral part), 2 – Orbital septum, 3 – Superior tarsus, 4 – Lateral palpebral ligament, 5 – Raphe of lateral palpebral ligament, 6 – Inferior tarsus, 7 – Orbital fat, 8 - Inferior oblique muscle, 9 – Lacrimal sac, 10 – Medial palpebral ligament,11 – Infratrochlear nerve, 12 – Supratrochlear nerve, 13 – Tendon of superior oblique muscle, 14 - Supraorbital nerve, 15 – Levator plapebrae superioris muscle. (Sketch is made on the base Sinelnikov R.D., Sinelnikov JA.R., Sinelnikov A. JA.: Atlas of human anatomy, Novaja volna, Moscow, 2007-2010).

The superior lateral corner forms a joint of the superior and the lateral orbital wall. In the posterior third of this corner there is a superior orbital fissure (*fissura orbitalis superior).* It connects the orbit with the medial cranial fossa (*fossa cranii media).* The fissure is bordered by the lateral side of the sphenoid bone body, as well as the lesser and greater wings of the same bone. The fissure is 18-20 mm long. The width of its medial, wider part varies and in most cases it is 8 – 10 mm. There are many arteries, veins and nerves passing through the superior orbital fissure. The following vessels and nerves pass through the medial, wider space of the fissure: the superior and the inferior terminal branch of oculomotor nerve, nasociliary nerve, abducens nerve, sympathetic branch to ciliary ganglion, and sometimes inferior ophthalmic vein Through the lateral, narrower space of the fissure pass: trochlear nerve, frontal nerve, lacrimal nerve as well as superior ophthalmic vein and anastomic branch of middle meningeal artery for the lacrimal artery (*ramus anastomaticus cum a.lacrimalis).*

The superior medial corner of the orbit forms a connection of its superior and medial wall. Around the centre of this orbital corner are two small round openings, anterior and posterior ethmoidal foramen. Small narrow ducts start from those openings connecting the eye cavity and the anterior cranial fossa i.e., the nasal cavity. Through the ethmoid openings and ducts pass the same-called arteries *(a.ethmoidalis anterior et posterior),* lateral branches of ophthalmic artery and the same-called nerves *(n.ethmoidalis anterior et posterior),* representing the branches of nasociliary nerve.

The inferior lateral corner of the orbit is located at the joint of its inferior and lateral wall. In the posterior three quarters of this corner the inferior orbital fissure is located. The inferior orbital fissure *(fissura orbitalis inferior)* connects the orbit with the infratemporal and the pterygopalatine fossa. The fissure is bordered by the body of the maxilla and the orbital side of the greater wing of the sphenoid bone. The medial margin of the inferior orbital fissure is formed by the orbital side of the body of the maxilla. This margin has a notch in the central part representing the beginning of the infraorbital grove. Through the inferior orbital fissure pass infraorbital artery and nerve, zygomatic nerve and the anastomotic veins which connect the eye cavity veins and the veins of the pterygoid plexus.

The inferior medial corner forms a joint of the inferior and the medial orbital wall. The upper opening of the nasolacrimal canal is located at the anterior end of this corner. The nasolacrimal canal *(canalis nasolacrimalis)* is formed by three bones: the maxilla, the lacrimal bone and the inferior nasal concha. It is around 10 mm long, 3 – 5 mm wide and it runs obliquely downwards, to the back and slightly medially. The nasolacrimal duct has the superior and the inferior opening. The superior opening is quite at the anterior end of the inferior medial corner of the orbit. The inferior opening of the canal is located immediately under the vault of the inferior nasal meatus.

1.4. Orbital Apex

The apex of the orbit (Figures 1, 2) is turned backwards and medially, and it consists of the anterior orbital opening of the optic canal. The optic canal *(canalis opticus)* connects the orbit and the medial cranial cavity *(fossa cranii media),* and it serves as a passage for the optic nerve and the ophthalmic artery, which is located in the canal below the nerve. The optic canal has two openings: anterior – orbital, and posterior – endocranial. From the orbital opening the canal runs obliquely backwards, medially and upwards. It is approximately cylindrical, most frequently 8-10 mm long, and 4-5 mm wide. The walls of the optic canal are formed by the anterior and the posterior root of the lesser wing and the lateral side of the sphenoid bone body. In the region of the orbital apex the common annular tendon is affixed *(anulus tendineus communis – the annulus of Zinn).* The common annular tendon represents the posterior, common insertion of the four rectus muscles of the eyeball.

1.5. Orbital Periosteum (Periorbit)

The orbital periosteum is a thin connective membrane covering the bony walls of the orbit and it is mainly easily peeled off. In the region of the lacrimal fossa the eye cavity periosteum is divided into the medial and lateral leaf. The medial leaf covers the floor of the lacrimal fossa. The lateral leaf forms a bridgelike crossing from the anterior to the posterior lacrimal crest. Thus the lacrimal sac lies in the duplicated periosteum of the orbit. Below the lacrimal fossa the periorbit continues into the periosteum of the nasolacrimal duct. In the region of the superior orbital fissure the periosteum covers the lateral, narrower space of the fissure and is fused hard with dura mater. In the region of the inferior orbital fissure the periosteum covers and closes the fissure. This part of the periosteum also contains smooth muscular fibers making the thin orbital Miller's muscle. This muscle is innervated by the sympathetic nerve fibers. The effect of this orbital muscle still remains unexplained. The general opinion was that the muscle represses the eyeball frontward causing exophthalmus. With the damage to the neck sympaticus (Burger's centre C8-Th1), ptosis, miosis and enophthalmos occur due to the palsy of the orbital muscles (Claude Bernard Horner syndrome). However, it is hard to believe that palsy of the thin orbital Miller's muscle can be the cause of enophthalmos.

1.6. Orbital Relations

The orbit is open and through its walls, corners and fissures it is connected to many important surrounding structures (Figures 1-10).

The superior wall, or the orbital roof, is also the floor for the anterior cranial fossa, and thus it is approximated to the brain membranes and the lower side of the frontal lobe of the brain. In the superior orbital wall there is more or less developed frontal sinus, often with anterior ethmoid cells.

In most people the frontal sinus corresponds to the anteromedial part of the orbital roof and its apex most often reaches supraorbital incisure. However, in around 14% of the cases, most often bilaterally, the frontal sinuses divide two leaves of the compact bone tissue in the orbital roof forming the supraorbital extension. The expansion of the frontal sinus in anteroposterior direction in the orbital roof is usually shallow and occasionally disturbed by the penetration of certain ethmoid cells into the horizontal part of the frontal bone. These ethmoid cells are called supplementary frontal sinuses and they are completely closed bony cavities with special drain ducts or openings by which they are connected to the middle or superior nasal meatus. Data in the literature regarding the frequency of supplementary frontal sinuses is quite diverse.

The inferior wall, or the orbital floor, is related to the maxillary sinus. In about 20% of people, the ethmoid cells spreading laterally and downwards, can more or less penetrate into the roof of the maxillary sinus.

The lateral wall of the orbit is the thickest and the firmest. Its anterior two thirds are in relation to the temporal fossa and its content (temporal muscle, deep temporal blood vessels and nerves). The posterior third of the lateral wall is in relation to the middle cranial fossa.

The medial orbital wall is in relation to the upper part of the nasal cavity and paranasal sinuses. The anterior part of the medial wall (the frontal process of the maxilla and the anterior part of the lacrimal bone) is directly related to the nasal cavity, middle nasal meatus and the lower part of the frontal sinus. There the lacrimal fossa is also located. The middle, biggest part of the medial orbital wall is in relation to the ethmoid cells, which are separating the orbit from the nasal cavity at the level of the superior and middle nasal meatus. The ethmoid cells are classified into the anterior, which open into the middle nasal meatus, and the posterior, which open into the superior nasal meatus. The lateral wall of the ethmoid labyrinth separating the ethmoid cells from the orbit, is made of a very thin bone leaf. The posterior part of the medial wall of the orbit is in relation to the sphenoid sinus, which can be very closely related to the optic canal and the nerve. The analysis of the orbital relations indicates that three out of four orbital walls (superior, inferior and medial) have very close relations to the paranasal sinuses, so the sinuses can also be referred as the "periorbital sinuses."

However, in children the relations of the orbit and the paranasal sinuse are not that close because the sinuses generally develop gradually during childhood. After puberty, around the age of twenty, they become fully developed. The ethmoid sinus consists of the anterior and posterior ethmoid cells which occupy the ethmoid labyrinth. In newborns this sinus is formed by several small and shallow recesses which develop in all directions during the first year of life. In the second year the ethmoid cells penetrate deeper into the ethmoid labyrinth coming into close relation with the medial wall of the orbit. The frontal sinu*s* is formed by invagination of one of the anterior ethmoid cells between the frontal bone leaves. This happens already at the age of two, but usually stays in the initial stage until the age of five. Around the age of five the frontal sinuses are usually the size of a small almond and are located in the vicinity of the superior medial corner of the orbit. From the age of five to the age of ten the frontal sinuses gradually develop and expand into the frontal bone, and they are squeezed in the space between the orbits. In young children the frontal sinus and the orbit are only related through the lateral sinus wall. After the age of ten the frontal sinus reaches the orbital roof and around the age of fifteen it starts expanding in the orbital roof, so the contacts between the sinuses and the orbit are considerably wider. In the period from the age of fifteen to the age of twenty the frontal sinuses mainly acquire the characteristics of the sinuses in adults and form definite relations with the orbit. The maxillary sinus represents quite developed cavity even in newborns, and it resembles the sagittally positioned trilateral pyramid with the apex directed frontward and the base directed backwards. After birth the maxillary sinus develops in all directions.

The maxillary sinus in children and in adults is related to the orbit through the superior wall which is very thin (0.5 – 1 mm). The relations between the maxillary sinus and the orbital floor are formed already during the first year of life. At the age of two, the maxillary sinus is expanded laterally, albeit more backwards than frontwards, so it still fails to reach the infraorbital canal. At the age of four and five the maxillary sinus has been already sufficiently developed laterally and passes under the entire inferior wall of the infraorbital canal, thus simultaneously forming considerably wider contact with the orbital floor. Around the age of seven the maxillary sinus reaches the zygomatic process of the maxilla, so the entire orbital floor is related to the maxillary sinus, from which it separates by a thin bony wall.

During the postnatal development the sphenoid sinus undergoes two stages. In the first stage, until the age of four or six, the sinus is in the so-called Bertin's ossicle, which adheres to the anterior side of the body of the sphenoid bone. This initial sphenoid sinus is quite far from the posterior part of the medial wall of the orbit. Between the age of four and six the initial sphenoid sinuses are expanded into the body of the sphenoid bone and already around the age of six the lateral wall of the sinus becomes thin, so the sinus comes into the close relation with the medial wall of the orbit and the medial end of the superior orbital fissure.

The sphenoid sinus then develops upwards and backwards and approaches the optic canal, so the wall between the sphenoid sinus and the optic canal can become thin as a paper. Only around the age of twenty, is the development of the sphenoid sinus is completed and it acquires the dimensions and proportion of the sinus in adults.

1.7. Eyelids (Palpebrae)

The eyelids (Figures 3, 4) are the skin folds that cover the bony eye cavity anteriorly, thus protecting its content. It is by constant movement that they distribute tears and provide moisturizing and watering of the cornea. An eye has an upper and lower eyelid *(palpebra superior and palpebra interior).* The upper eyelid is twice wider than the lower one. At the borderline between the upper eyelid and the forehead skin there is an arched protuberance called the eyebrow (*supercilium)* covered with obliquely inserted hairs. The eyebrow protuberance is formed of a fat tissue and of superficial, subcutaneous muscles, *(m. occipitofrontalis, m.depressor supercilii and m.corrugator supercilii).* These muscles are innerved through the branches of the facial nerve (*n. facialis).* The eyelids have the anterior and posterior side and the free margin. The free margins of the upper and lower eyelid limit the interpalpebral opening. The anterior side of the eyelids (*facies anterior palpebrarum)* is coated with thin skin. In the middle of the anterior side of the upper eyelid, especially when it is raised, the superior palpebral sulcus is visible, concave downwards. This sulcus represents the borderline between the lower solid tarsal and the upper flexible orbital part of the eyelid. The superior palpebral sulcus is formed by insertion of tendon fibers of levator palpebrae superioris muscle on the deep side of the skin. At the anterior side of the lower eyelid the inferopr palpebral sulcus is visible with concavity turned upwards. The posterior side of the eyelid *(facies posterior palpebrarum)* is concave and covered with smooth and pink conjunctiva *(tunica conjunctiva palpebrarum).* Vertical, yellowish, mutually parallel stripes are transparent through the conjunctiva, which are formed by extended Meibomius' tarsal glands. The free margins of the eyelids are divided by a short, conical, lacrimal papilla (*papilla lacrimalis)* in two unequal parts – lateral and medial. The lateral part of the free margin is considerably longer and it occupies seven eights of the margin. It is also considerably wider, around 2-3 mm, and two borders can be differentiated – anterior and posterior. The anterior palpebral borders (*limbi palpebrales anteriores)* are rounded and have eyelashes *(cilia)*, which are inserted obliquely in two or three rows. Their task, as well as that of the eyelid, is to protect the cornea and the conjunctiva. The posterior palpebral borders *(limbi palpebrales posteriores)* are sharp and signify the transmission of the eyelid skin into the conjunctiva. Immediately in front of the posterior limbs, i.e., behind the eyelashes, a series of around 20 to 30 spot openings of Meibomius' tarsal glands are visible. The medial part of the free margin of the eyelid is considerably shorter and narrower than the lateral one and has no eyelashes, and therefore no borders can be differentiated on it. The medial parts of the free margins of the eyelids form the so-called lacrimal lake *(lacus lacrimalis).*

The palpebral opening *(rima palpebrarum)* has changeable shape and size. When the eye is open, rima palpebrarum has almond-like or oval shape. If the eye is closed, the palpebral opening is narrow and slightly concave upwards. When the eye is open, the upper eyelid with its free margin covers around 0.5 to 1 mm of the superior margin of the cornea, while the free margin of the lower eyelid lies on the inferior margin of the cornea. Therefore, when the eye is open the entire cornea is visible in the palpebral opening with the exception of its upper part. When the eye is closed the lower eyelid raises covering the inferior margin of the cornea for about 1 mm. The upper eyelid descends until meeting with the lower one and it covers almost the entire cornea, except for its lowest part. So, when the eye is closed the centre of the cornea is behind the upper eyelid.

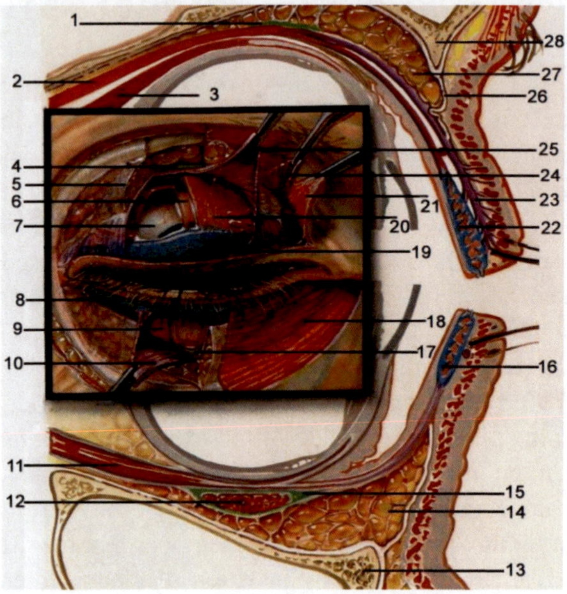

Figure 4. Structure of the upper and the lower eyelid (Zide B.M., Jelks G.W., Surgical anatomy of the orbit, Raven Press, New York, 1985). 1 and 4 – Whitnall's ligament, 2 – Levator palpebreae superioris muscle, 3 – Superior rectus muscle, 5 and 26 – Orbital septum, 6 and 9 – Conjunctiva, 7 – Eye ball, 8 and 16 – Inferior tarsus, 10 – Horner's muscle of the lower eyelid, 11 –Inferior rectus muscle, 12 – Inferior oblique muscle, 13 – Inferior orbital margin, 14 and 27 – Orbital fat, 15 and 17- Lockwood ligament, 18 and 24 – Orbicularis oculi muscle, 19 and 22 – Superior tarsus, 20 – Müller muscle, 21 – Upper eyelid skin, 23 and 25 – Aponeurosis of the levator palpebre superioris muscle, 28 – Superior orbital margin.

The palpebral opening forms ocular angles on both of its ends. Lateral ocular angle *(angulus oculi lateralis),* formed by the lateral parts of the eyelid free margins, is sharp, while the medial ocular angle *(angulus oculi medialis)* is rounded. In Indo-European nations the palpebral opening has a horizontal position. If the lateral angle is higher in comparison to the medial one, that represents Mongoloid position of palpebral opening. If, on the other hand, the lateral ocular angle is lower in comparison to the medial one, then it is a Negroid position.

In children, in the area of medial angle, the vertical semilunar skin fold, laterally concave may occur, which is called palpebronasal fold or epicanthus *(plica palpebronasalis seu epicanthus).* This fold disappears with time, however, it is permanently present in Mongolians.

From the lateral ocular angle, 5 to 7 mm long lateral commissure of the eyelids *(commissura palpebrarum lateralis)* runs horizontally to the lateral margin of the orbital aperture. From the medial ocular angle, the medial commissure of the eyelids *(commissura palpebrarum medialis)* spreads towards the medial margin of the orbital aperture, which is projected by the medial palpebral ligament *(lig. palpebrale mediale).*

The thin skin covers the anterior side of the eyelids. Its deep layer is connected to the orbital septum *(septum orbitale)* by thin connective fibers. In the lateral region of the free margins of the eyelids, bearing the eyelashes, the skin is slightly thickened. Sebaceous glands open next to the eyelash on the anterior palpebral borders, and their infection causes external stye.

The subcutaneous layer of the eyelids is formed by a very loose connective tissue, almost without fat tissue, which enables mild skin folding which is necessary for moving the eyelids.

The layer of striated muscles is formed by the orbicularis oculi muscle and the levator of the upper eyelid. The orbicularis oculi muscle *(m.orbicularis oculi)* is part of the subcutaneous mimic head muscles. It is a thin, flat muscle having an elliptic form, which lies beneath the skin of the bony entry opening of the orbit, as well as in the eyelids. With regard to the insertions and the function, the orbicular ocular muscle has four parts: orbital, palpebral, lacrimal and ciliary. Orbital part is the peripheral part of the muscle, surrounding its palpebral part, i.e., the bony aperture of the orbit. Elliptic fibers of the orbital part are attached to the frontal process of the maxilla, i.e., to the anterior lacrimal crest and the medial palpebral ligament. Palpebral part is directly beneath the skin of the upper and the lower eyelid, i.e., on the inner side of orbital part, with which it continues without a clear border. Semicircular muscular fibers are inserted medially to the medial palpebral ligament, and laterally – to the lateral palpebral ligament. Lacrimal part is a short, flat triangular muscle which lies at the posterior side of the lacrimal sac. Ciliary part consists of thin fibers around the eyelashes root. The orbicularis oculi muscle is innervated by facial nerve ie. with its *rr.temporales* and *rr.zygomatici.* The orbicularis oculi muscle has various functions due its complex composition. By a joint contraction of orbital and palpebral parts the eyelids are firmly shut. Palpebral part of the muscle presses the eyelids against the eyeball mildly shutting the eyelids, for example, during sleeping or blinking. Lacrimal part of the muscle empties the lacrimal sac pushing the tears through the lacrimal ducts. Patients suffering from the paralysis of the facial nerve cannot shut the eye, leaving the eye always open *(lagophthalmus).* Due to the loss of tonus of the orbicularis ocular muscle the lower eyelid is detached from the eyeball *(ectropion)* and the tears drop over the eyelid margin onto the cheek *(epiphora).* The levator palpebrae superior muscle *(m. levator palpebrae superioris)* is just beneath the orbital roof and spreads from the apex of the orbit to the upper eyelid. The levator palpebrae superior muscle is affixed at the back in the area of the orbital apex, immediately above the annulus of Zinn and the optic canal, i.e., on the lower side of the lesser wing of the sphenoid bone. The flat muscle spreads obliquely frontward and laterally, immediately beneath the orbital roof and the frontal nerve, and above the superior rectus muscle. The levator palpebrae superior muscle covers almost entirely the superior rectus muscle, except its lateral margin. In front of the eyeball equator the muscle gradually bends downwards and turns into a very wide terminal tendon which, with its central part, enters the upper eyelid; and the side extensions, lateral and medial ones, affix onto the corresponding bony orbital wall. The central part of the terminal tendon of levator palpebrae superioris muscle divides in two laminas. The superficial lamina *(lamina superficialis)* is more developed, penetrates orbital septum and orbicularis oculi muscle and is annexed to the deep side of the upper eyelid skin in the region of the superior palpebral sulcus. The deep lamina *(lamina profunda)* is less developed and is annexed onto the superior convex margin and onto the anterior side of the superior tarsus. The lateral side extension of the terminal tendon of the lervator palpebrae superioris muscle spreads laterally, between the orbital and the palpebral part of the lacrimal gland and is attached to the lateral wall of the orbit, along the posterior margin of the frontozygomatic suture. The lateral extension is about 2-3 mm wide, and it is penetrated by the excretory ducts of the lacrimal gland. The medial side extension of the terminal tendon of the levator palpebrae superioris muscle is attached to the upper end of the posterior lacrimal crest of the lacrimal bone. The levator palpebrae superioris muscle is innerved by the branches of the oculomotor nerve, and therefore when the nerve is paralyzed the upper eyelid is lowered and cannot be lifted actively. The levator palpebrae superior muscle, by pulling the upper eyelid upwards, opens the eye. In the waking state this muscle is almost always in function and it opens the eye again after every blink. Its wide and solid lateral side extension, which is penetrated by the excretory ducts of the lacrimal gland, has an important function. This extension distributes the tears throughout the entire length of the upper vault of the conjunctiva, thus providing the moisturizing of the entire cornea.

The fibrous layer of the eyelids consists of the orbital septum, the superior and the inferior tarsus and the lateral and the medial palpebral ligament.

The orbital septum *(septum orbitale)* is approximately rectangular fibrous plate which is attached to the bony margin of the orbital aperture, while in the central part, i.e., in the region of palpebral opening, it displays a wide horizontal slit. The orbital septum is a peripheral and flexible part of the fibrous layer of the eyelid. The superior and the inferior tarsus form a central, solid, inflexible region of the fibrous layer of the eyelid. The orbital septum on the superior margin of the orbit passes over two incisures *(incisura supraorbitalis, incisura frontalis)* transforming them into osteofibrous openings for the passing of blood vessels and nerves. The medial part of the orbital septum is attached to the posterior lacrimal crest of the lacrimal bone, i.e., behind the lacrimal sac. The central part of the orbital septum is very thin and covers the anterior sides of the superior and the inferior tarsus. The orbital septum and the wide terminal tendon of levator palpebrae superioris muscle form a solid fibrous septum between the two well-restricted fascial spaces in the upper eyelid – preseptal and pretarsal space. The preseptal space is limited by: at the front – palpebral part of the orbicularis oculi muscle, at the back and upward – orbital septum, and at the back and downward – terminal tendon of levator palpebrae superioris muscle. The preseptal space contains a very small quantity of the fat tissue, and also the superior arterial palpebral arch *(arcus palpebralis superior)* in the lower part. The pretarsal space is limited: at the front – by the terminal tendon of levator palpebrae superioris muscle, at the back and upwards – by superior tarsal muscle, and at the back and downwards – by tarsus superior. The pretarsal space frequently contains the arterial peripheral palpebral arch, and in the lateral part of it, the palpebral part of the lacrimal gland is located.

The superior tarsus *(tarsus superior)* and the inferior tarsus *(tarsus inferior)* are solid, middle inflexible structures of the fibrous layer of the upper and the lower eyelid. Both tarsus have a semilunar shape whose horizontal margin lies in the free margin of the corresponding eyelid, while their peripheral margin is convex. The anterior side of the tarsus is convex, the posterior side is concave and corresponds to the eyeball concavity, from which the tarsus is separated only by the conjunctiva. The lateral and the medial palpebral ligament, which connect the tarsus with the lateral and the medial margin of the orbital aperture, start from the ends of both tarsus. The superior tarsus, with a maximum width of 10 mm, is twice wider than the inferior tarsus. The tarsus are formed by a compact connective tissue which gives the shape to the eyelid. This tissue also contains special Meibomius' sebaceous tarsal glands, 30-40 in the upper eyelid, and 20-30 in the lower one. The tarsal glands are elongated, mutually aligned parallel and vertical to the free margin of the eyelid. They spread almost along the entire width of the corresponding tarsus, and they are longer in the middle and shorter towards the ends of the tarsus. When the eyelid is twisted, the Meibomius' glands are transparent through the conjunctiva in the form of parallel brown stripes resembling the comb teeth. Vertical or slightly bent excretory ducts of the Meibomius' glands end in tiny openings aligned behind the eyelash, immediately in front of the posterior border of the free eyelid margin. The tarsal glands discharge sebum that covers the free margins of the eyelids preventing the spillage of the tears over the eyelid rim.

The lateral palpebral ligament *(lig. palpebrale laterale)* and the medial palpebral ligament *(lig. palpebrale mediale)* connect the lateral, i.e., the medial end of both tarsus with the lateral, i.e., the medial margin of the orbital aperure. The lateral palpebral ligament spreads horizontally from the lateral ends of the superior and the inferior tarsus to the lateral margin of the orbital aperture where it is attached immediately under the frontozygomatic suture. The medial palpebral ligament separates from the medial ends of the superior and the inferior tarsus and spreads horizontally towards the middle. On the medial end it divides into anterior and posterior band. The anterior band attaches to the anterior lacrimal crest in front of the lacrimal sac. The posterior band connects behind the lacrimal sac to the posterior lacrimal crest of the lacrimal bone. Medial ligament forms protuberance in the skin in the area of the internal palpebral commissure.

The layer of smooth eyelid muscles consists of thin tarsal muscles – superior and inferior, which are behind the orbital septum. The superior tarsal muscle *(m. tarsalis superior)* – Müller's muscle – is around 10 mm wide and spreads from the superior margin of the superior tarsus to the terminal tendon of levator palpebrae superioris muscle. The inferior tarsal muscle *(m. tarsalis inferior)* – Horner's muscle – is less developed than the upper one. It consists of straight vertical muscular fibers spreading from the inferior margin of the inferior tarsus to the palpebral extension of inferior rectus muscle and the inferior fornix of the conjunctiva. Both tarsal muscles are innerved by the sympathetic branches. With their tonus the superior and the inferior tarsal muscle maintain the normal width of palpebral opening.

The mucous membrane of the eyelids represents the deepest layer and it consists of a smooth, shiny and transparent tunic, conjunctiva - *tunica conjunctiva palpebrarum.* The conjunctiva is a thin, transparent and shiny membrane connecting the posterior side of the eyelids with the eyeball. The conjunctiva covers the posterior side of the upper and the lower eyelid, and then moves from the eyelids to the anterior part of the eyeball covering everything to the border of cornea *(limbus corneae).* When moving from the eyelid to the eyeball the conjunctiva bends forming the upper and the inferior fornix. When the eyes are closed, the conjunctiva forms a narrow cavity, called the conjunctival sac *(saccus conjunctivae),* which contains tears. The anterior wall of this sac is formed by palpebral conjunctiva, and the posterior wall is formed by the eyeball conjunctiva supplemented by the anterior side of the cornea. Conjunctival sac is always a very thin cavity, but after the enucleation of the eyeball, a space emerges in which it is possible to place the eye prosthesis.

A semilunar conjunctival fold *(plica semilunaris conjunctivae)* is located in the medial corner of the eye and it has the shape of an elongated vertically positioned crescent, with concavity towards the cornea border. This fold, together with the medial ends of free margins of the upper and the lower eyelid forms a lacrimal lake *(lacus lacrimalis)*. The semilunar conjunctival fold represents a rudimentary remnant of the third palpebra and arguably has no significance for the eye movements. The lacrimal caruncle *(caruncula lacrimalis)* is a cone-shaped convexity 3-5 mm in size, which is located in the lacrimal lake in the medial corner of the eye. The top of the lacrimal caruncle is positioned laterally downwards and it is covered by the lower eyelid and can be seen only after the eyelid had been pulled down and laterally. The caruncle has the skin-like composition, so it contains hairs and sebaceous glands. It is protruded by the fat tissue located inside subconjunctival connective tissue.

1.8. Lacrimal Apparatus (Apparatus Lacrimalis)

The lacrimal apparatus (Figure 5) consists of the lacrimal gland, which secretes the tears, and the excretory part. The tears flow through the excretory ducts of the lacrimal gland into the upper conjunctival fornix, thus constantly keeping the conjunctiva and the anterior surface of the cornea moist, also rinsing conjunctival sac. By blinking, the eyelids evenly distribute the tears into all the areas of conjunctival sac.

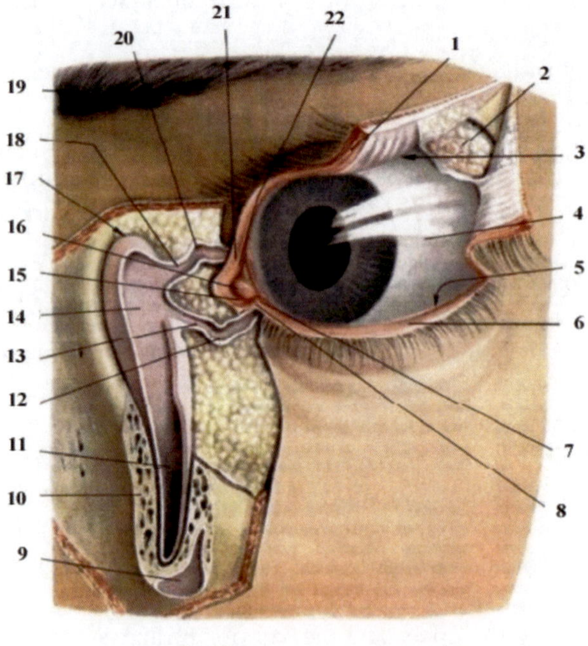

Figure 5. Lacrimal apparatus. 1 – Upper eyelid, 2 – Lacrimal gland, 3 – Superior conjunctival fornix, 4 – Bulbar conjunctiva 5 – Inferor conjunctival fornix, 6 – Lower eyelid, 7 – Lacrimal punctum, 8 – Lacrimal papilla, 9 – Maxillary sinus, 10 – Frontal process of maxilla, 11 – Nasolacrimal duct, 12 - Ampula canaliculi lacrimalis, 13 – Inferior lacrimal cnalicul. 14 – Lacrimal sac, 15 – Lacrimal lacus, 16 – Lacrimal caruncule, 17 – Fornix of lacrimal sac, 18 – Superior lacrimal canalicul, 19 – Supercilium, 20 – Ampula canaliculi lacrimalis. 21 – Lacrimal punctum, 22 – Lacrimal papilla (Sketch is made on the base Sinelnikov R. D., Sinelnikov JA. R., Sinelnikov A. JA.: Atlas of human anatomy, Novaja volna, Moscow, 2007-2010).

1.8.1. Lacrimal Gland (Glandula Lacrimalis)

The lacrimal gland is a secretory organ of the lacrimal apparatus. By the solid lateral extension of the terminal tendon of the upper eyelid levator muscle, the gland is divided in two unequal parts: orbital and palpebral. The orbital part (*pars orbitalis),* with dimensions 5x10x20 mm, is bigger than the palpebral one. It is located in the fossa of lacrimal gland *(fossa glandulae lacrimalis),* which is concave at the anterior-lateral corner of the orbital side of the frontal bone. The palpebral part (*pars palpebralis)* of the lacrimal gland is located below the orbital part. It is considerably smaller and makes only one quarter to one third of the gland. The palpebral part is located in the lateral area of the upper eyelid.

The orbital part of the lacrimal gland has three to five excretory ducts penetrating the lateral side extension of the terminal tendon of levator palbebre superioris muscle. The excretory ducts spread downwards, pass through the palpebral part of the lacrimal gland and on their way receive numerous short ducts from the lateral half of the palpebral part. From the medial half of the palpebral part, 3 to 9 ducts exit separately. All excretory ducts, the total number 8-12, are vertical and parallel. They irrigate in the lateral part of the superior fornix of the conjunctiva.

1.8.2. Excretory Part of the Lacrimal Apparatus

Blinking distributes the tears from the superior fornix of the conjunctiva along the entire conjunctival sac. Tears are then collected in the lacrimal lake. From the lacrimal lake, through the lacrimal points (*puncta lacrimalia*), which are located on the top of the lacrimal papilla, the tears are sucked into the lacrimal ducts (*canaliculi lacrimalis*), which guide them to the lacrimal sac *(sacus lacrimalis).* From the lacrimal sac the tears outflow through the nasolacrimal duct *(ductus nasolacrimalis)* into the inferior nasal meatus. The lacrimal sack is a cylindrical formation, it is located in its bone fossa at the anterior end of the medial wall of the orbit. Its superior, closed end, fornix of the lacrimal sac *(fornix sacci lacrimalis),* usually is located above the medial palpebral ligament, or is in line with the ligament. The inferior end of the lacrimal sack corresponds to the level of the inferior wall of the orbit, at the same time representing the superior opening of the nasolacrimal duct. The height of the lacrimal sac is 12 – 15 mm, its anteroposterior diameter is 6 -7 mm, transverse diameter is around 4 – 5 mm. The anterior side of the lacrimal sac is covered by the skin of the medial palpebral commissure, fibers of orbicularis oculi muscle and anterior band of medial palpebral ligament. The skin is very thin and movable. The anterior band of the medial palpebral ligament divides the anterior side of the lacrimal sac into two unequal parts. The upper part is smaller and reaches 1 to 2 mm above the ligament. The lower part is much bigger and is the site where incision of the lacrimal sac can be performed. This part of the sac is covered with loose fibers of orbicularis oculi muscle, it is easily stretched and bulged out due to a high pressure in the sac (pus, etc.). Medial palpebral ligament is a signpost for accessing the lacrimal sac. Tumefactions which are located below this ligament almost always belong to the lacrimal sac (e.g.,, purulent processes). The tumefactions above the ligament are mainly caused by the changes in the paranasal sinuses and cranium (mucocela, meningocela). The posterior side of the lacrimal sac lies on the posterior band of the medial palpebral ligament, lacrimal part of orbicularis oculi muscle and orbital septum, separating the sac from the orbital fat. The lateral side of the lacrimal sac is surrounded by the fork of the medial palpebral ligament and is in relation with the lacrimal ducts. A common lacrimal duct goes through the upper area flowing into the lacrimal sac. The medial side of the lacrimal sac lies at the bottom of the lacrimal fossa, which is covered by periosteum. The medial or the nasal side of this cavity has very variable and complex relations with the nasal cavity and the paranasal sinuses.

The nasolacrimal duct represents the inferior extension of the lacrimal sac, mostly hidden in the bone canal with the same name. Its walls are made of: maxilla, lacrimal bone and the inferior nasal concha. The tears flow from the lacrimal sac into the inferior nasal meatus along the fibro-mucous nasolacrimal duct.

1.9. Eyeball Fascia (Fascia Bulbi) or Tenon's Capsule

Tenon's capsule or the eyeball membrane *(fascia seu vagina bulbi)* represents a solid fibrous membrane covering the posterior four fifths or five sixths of the eyeball. Extensions spreading from Tenon's capsule create the fascial membranes of the orbital extrabulbar muscles, These fascial membranes, in the anterior area of the orbit and the orbital aperture, send the fascial extensions towards the walls of the orbit, the eyelids and the conjuctival vaults (1, 2, 3, 5). Tenon's capsule, like the sclera, resembles a segment of a hollow ball spreading from the corneal limb backwards to the optic nerve opening at the posterior part of the sclera. The capsule is the thickest around the eyeball equator, gradually thinning as moving backwards. The anterior part of Tenon's capsule is firmly affixed to the anterior part of the sclera around the corneal limb, while the posterior part adheres with the dural membrane of the optical nerve and the surrounding part of the sclera. The external surface of Tenon's capsule, facing the bony orbital walls, is convex and covered with the eyeball conjunctiva at the front, and with the fat tissue of the orbit at the back. Six muscles that move the eyeball pass through the anterior part of the Tenon's capsule. The fascial extensions spreading from Tenon's capsule, envelope the tendons of the rectus and oblique ocular muscles in the area of the muscular openings, all the way to their annexes at the sclera. The fascial extensions, going backwards and covering the bodies of the mentioned muscles that move the eyeball, also spread from Tenon's capsule. Tenon's subfascial space is elongated frontward around the muscular tendons forming extensions or diverticulums around them. The fascial extensions spread from the muscular fascia in the anterior orbital area, as well as in the orbital aperture area, connecting the muscular fascia and indirectly also Tenon's capsule, to the bony orbital walls, the eyelids and the conjunctival fornices. The intermuscular septa between the inferior oblique and the inferior rectus muscle form the inferior transversal suspensory ligament – the Lockwood's ligament. Similarly, the septa spreading along the upper part of the levator palpebrae superioris muscle, or surrounding it, form the superior transversal ligament – Whitnall's ligament [2, 5]. The fascial extensions towards the bony orbital walls spread from the fascias of all four rectus muscles and the superior oblique muscle, as well as from the fascia of the upper eyelid levator muscle, connecting those fasciae and Tenon's capsule to the corresponding eye cavity wall. These connections and the surrounding fat tissue affix Tenon's capsule, which is the basis for its functioning. Namely, the affixed Tenon's capsule allows the function of orbital, extrabulbar muscles and prevents its moving backwards during muscle contraction. The eyeball rotates in Tenon's capsule concavity as the head of the ball joint in a motionless cup [1, 2]. Out of these fascial extensions the most important ones are those spreading from the fascia of the lateral and the medial rectus muscle going towards the lateral, i.e., medial wall of the orbit. The extension of the fascia of the lateral rectus muscle spreads obliquely to laterally and connects to the lateral wall of the orbit just above the insertion of lateral palpebral ligament. The extension of the fascia of the medial rectus muscle is less developed and spreads obliquely medially and frontward and it is fixed at the upper end of posterior lacrimal crest, behind the lacrimal sac. The fascial extensions towards the upper eyelid start from the fascial membrane of the upper eyelid levator muscle, and, towards the lower eyelid, from the membrane of the inferior rectus muscle. The fascial extensions for the upper eyelid and the fascial extensions mutually connecting the muscular fasciae of upper palpebre levator muscle and rectus superior muscle allow synergetic lifting of the upper eyelid and the eyeball when looking upwards. The fascial extension of rectus inferior muscle separates from the anterior part of this muscle membrane, spreading frontward, entering the lower eyelid where it is fixed along the inferior margin of the inferior tarsus. This fascial extension pulls the lower eyelid downwards at contraction of rectus inferior muscle, i.e., at looking downwards. The fascial extensions towards the conjunctival fornices also spread from the muscular fasciae. Their role is to stretch the conjunctiva preventing its folding.

1.10. Retrobulbar Space (Spatium Retrobulbare) and Parabulbar Space (Spatium Parabulbare)

In clinical practice the orbit is most often divided in three spaces: peribulbar, parabulbar and retrobulbar. This division does not include the eyeball. The peribulbar space is a narrow space immediately surrounding the entire eyeball. The parabulbar space is a wide area of the orbit located above, below, laterally and medially from the eyeball. This space spreads from the orbital septum backwards to the frontal section which passes through the posterior pole of the eyeball.

The retrobulbar space includes the entire area of the orbit behind the eyeball, i.e., behind the mentioned frontal section. This space is divided by four rectus muscles into intraconal and extraconal space. The four rectus muscles, fixed in the area of the orbital apex at the annulus of Zinn, encircle the eyeball. The middle area of the retrobulbar space, located within the muscle cone is called the intraconal space, and the peripheral area, around the rectus muscles, extraconal space. In the retrobulbar and the parabulbar space, the lacrimal gland, orbital muscles, arteries, veins, lymphatic system, nerves, and orbital fat tissue are all located.

1.11. Orbital Muscles

The orbital muscles include seven striated muscles: the upper eyelid levator muscle (*m. levator palpebrae superioris),* four rectus muscles (*m. rectus superior, inferior, lateralis et medialis)* and two oblique muscles (*m. obliquus superior et inferior)* (Figures 2, 6, 7). All these muscles are thin, fleshy stripes. The extensions, forming the fascial membranes for all seven muscles, spread from Tenon's fascial capsule. Near the muscular openings on Tenon's capsule, at the front, these fascial membranes are somewhat thicker; going backwards they become thinner resulting in very thin membranes at the back. Upper eyelid levator muscle raises the upper eyelid. Four straight and two oblique muscles move the eyeball and therefore, in clinical medicine, they are referred to as the "bulbomotor muscles."

A detailed description of the upper eyelid levator was previously given in the eyelids section.

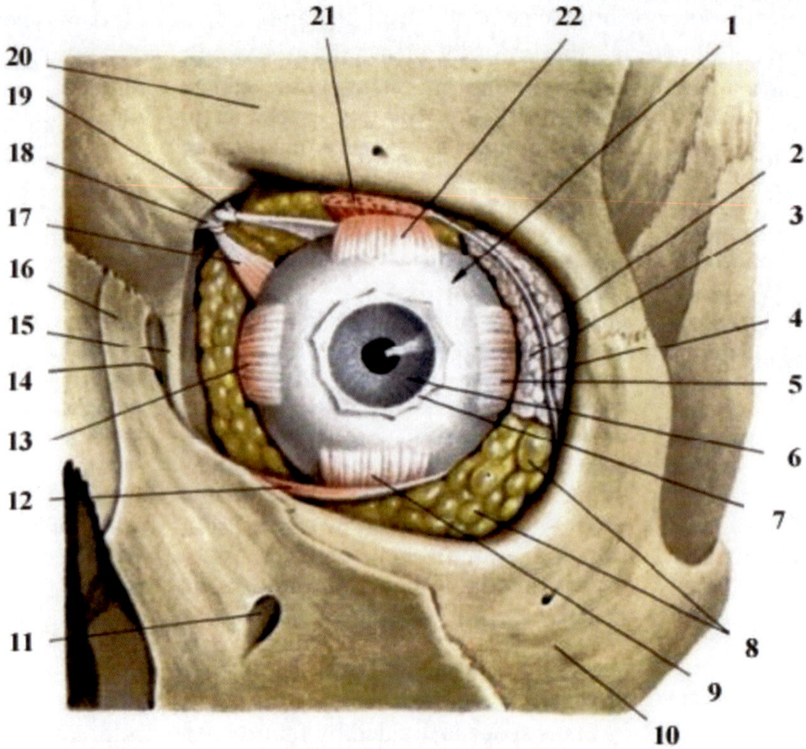

Figure 6. Extraocular muscles. 1 - Eye bulb, 2 – Orbital paret of lacrimal gland, 3 – Palpebral part of lacrimal gland, 4 – Deep lamina of levator palpebrea superioris muscle, 5 – Lateral rectus muscle, 6 – Cornea, 7 – Bulbar conjunctiva, 8 – Orbital fat, 9 – Inferior rectus muscle, 10 – Zygomatic bone, 11 - Infraorbital foramen, 12 – Inferior oblique muscle, 13 – Medial rectus muscle, 14 – Nasolacrimal canal, 15 – Posterior lacrimal crist. 16 – Frontal process, 17 – Superior oblique muscle, 18 – Trochlea, 19 - Synovial vagina of superior oblique muscle, 20 – Frontal bone, 21 – Levator palpebrea superioris muscle, 22 – Superior rectus muscle. (Sketch is made on the base Sinelnikov R. D., Sinelnikov JA.R., Sinelnikov A. JA.: Atlas of human anatomy, Novaja volna, Moscow, 2007-2010).

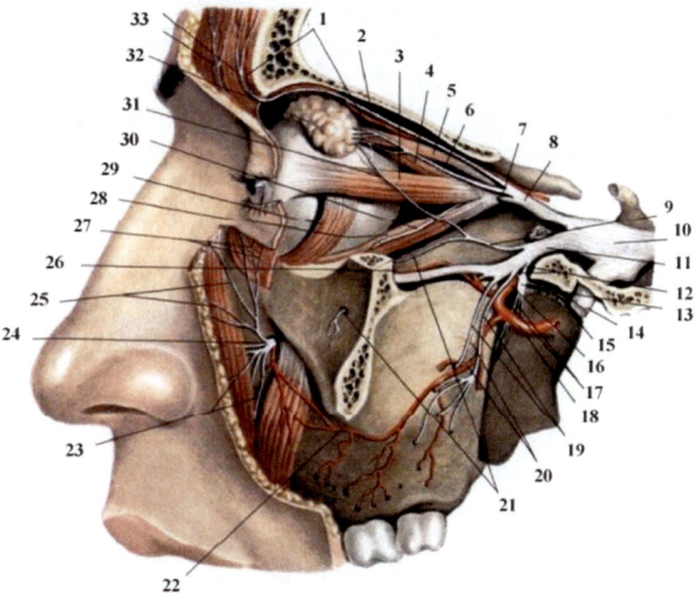

Figure 7. Content of orbit – lateral view. 1 – Supraorbital artery, 2 – Frontal nerve, 3 – Lateral rectus muscle, 4 – Superior rectus muscle, 5 – Levator palpebrea superioris muscle, 6 – Lacrimal nerve, 7 – Nasociliary nerve, 8 – Ophthalmic nerve, 9 – Zygomatic nerve, 10 – Trigeminal ganglion, 11 – Maxillary nerve, 12 – Ganglional branches, 13 Pterygoplatine ganglion, 14 – Mandibular nerve 15 – Nerve of pterygoid canal, 16 – Sphenopalatine artery, 17 – Greater and lesser palatine nerves, 18 – Maxillary artery, 19 - Posterior superior alveolar nerves, 20 – Posterior superior alveolar arteries, 21 – Zygomaticofacial branch of zygomatic nerve, 22 – Buccal artery, 23 – Labial branches of infraorbital nerve, 24 – Infraorbital nerve, 25 – Nasal branches of infraorbital nerve, 26 – Infraorbital artery, 27 – Palpebral branches of infraorbital nerve, 28 – Inferior rectus muscle, 29 – Inferior oblique muscle, 30 – Inferior division of oculomotor nerve, 31 - Communicating branch with zygomatic nerve, 32 - Lacrimal gland, 33 – Medial and lateral branches of supraorbital artery (Sketch is made on the base Sinelnikov R. D., Sinelnikov JA. R., Sinelnikov A. JA.: Atlas of human anatomy, Novaja volna, Moscow, 2007-2010).

1.11.1. Rectus Muscles

The eyeball has four rectus muscles: superior, inferior, lateral and medial. All four rectus muscles are connected at the back to the common annular tendon (annulus of Zinn). Through the cavity of this annulus optic nerve and ophthalmic artery enter the orbit, and laterally and below them – the final branches of the oculomotor nerve, abducens nerve and sympathetic branch for ciliary ganglion. The posterior ends of all four rectus muscles are fixed to the margin of the common annular tendon. The anterior ends of rectus muscles are annexed on the sclera, in front of the eyeball equator, along the spiral line close to the corneal margin. The annex of the internal rectus muscle is the closest to the corneal margin, at 5.5 mm distance. Then the spiral line spreads encompassing the annexes of the inferior rectus muscle which is at 6.5 mm distance from the corneal margin, and the external rectus muscle which is at 7 mm distance from the corneal margin, ending in the annex of the superior rectus muscle, which is at the greatest distance from the corneal limbus, i.e., at 7.7 mm. The anterior, terminal tendons of the rectus muscles after passing through Tenon's capsule are wrapped by cylindrical extensions of the capsule, which follow them all the way to the annex on the sclera. The terminal tendons are covered by the eyeball conjunctiva almost along their entire length. The rectus muscles are long and flat, somewhat wider at the anterior end. Their anterior ends perforate Tenon's capsule that forms fascial membranes for all the muscles of the eye cavity. The fascial extensions described above derive from those membranes connecting the extrabulbar muscles with the bony walls of the orbit, the eyelids and the conjunctival fornices. The rectus muscles are about 40 mm long, including the length of the tendon. The superior rectus muscle is a bit longer (around 41.8 mm) than others. The lateral rectus muscle obtains motor fibers from abducens nerve. Other three rectus muscles are innerved by oculomotor nerve.

1.11.2. Oblique Muscles

The eyeball has a superior and the inferior oblique muscle. The superior oblique muscle is the thinnest and the longest extraocular muscle. It starts directly above and medially from the anterior opening of the optic canal, spreading frontward, along the superior medial corner of the orbit. Its thin terminal tendon passes through the fibro-cartilaginous ring – trochlea, which is sometimes ossified. After the tendon passes through the trochlea, it suddenly turns backwards and laterally and ends fan-shaped under the superior rectus muscle on the eyeball, behind the equator.

The inferior oblique muscle is the shortest muscle of the extraocular muscles. The anterior medial end of the muscle is annexed on the inferior orbital wall directly behind and laterally from the lacrimal sac. The muscular body spreads obliquely backwards and laterally, over the orbital floor, passes under the anterior end of the inferior rectus muscle and turns upwards annexing behind the eyeball equator.

Inervation of the oblique muscles is diverse. The superior oblique muscle receives 3-4 branches from the trochlear nerve. The inferior oblique muscle is innervated by the terminal inferior branch of the oculomotor nerve.

1.11.3. Rectus and Oblique Muscles Function

The four rectus and the two oblique muscles of the eyeball move the eyeball in the concavity of Tenon's fascial capsule around the three axes of the eyeball: sagittal, vertical and horizontal. All three axes are mutually intersected in the so-called eyeball rotation point, which lies on the sagittal axis at around 13.5 mm behind the anterior pole of the eyeball. The vision line indicating the direction of the gaze is practically concurring with the sagittal axis. The superior rectus muscle pulls the anterior pole of the eyeball and cornea upwards (elevation). The inferior rectus muscle pulls the anterior pole of the eyeball downwards *(depressio)* and slightly medially *(adductio)*. The external rectus muscle, if the eyeball is in its primary position, pulls the anterior pole of the eyeball laterally *(abductio)*. If the eyeball is directed upwards, the muscle contributes to its further elevation, and vice versa, when looking downwards the muscle intensifies the eyeball depression. The internal rectus muscle, if the eyeball is in its primary position, pulls the anterior pole of the eyeball medially. The superior oblique muscle, when the eyeball is in its primary position, pulls its anterior pole and the cornea downwards and laterally simultaneously rotating it inwards. The inferior oblique muscle, when the eyeball is in its primary position, pulls its anterior pole and the cornea upwards and laterally at the same time rotating the eyeball laterally.

1.12. Orbital Arteries

The ophthalmic artery *(a. ophthalmica)* is the most important artery in the orbit. Its branches vascularize the eye and its accessory organs. In the bony inferior wall of the orbit there is the trunk of the infraorbital artery *(a. infraorbitalis).* Its branches supply certain orbital muscles and the lower eyelid (Figures 7, 8).

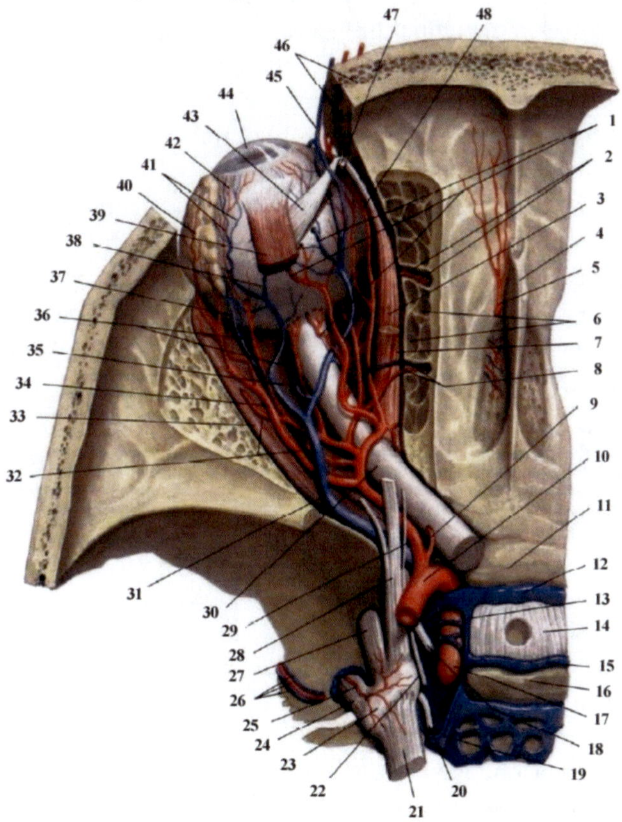

Figure 8. Orbital arteries and veins. 1-Posterior ciliari arteries and veins, 2-Anterior ethmoidal artery and vein, 3-superior oblique muscle, 4-Crista gally, 5-Anterior meningeal artery, 6-Ethmoidal cells, 7-Medial rectus muscle, 8 Posterior ethmoidal artery and vein, 9-Central artery of retina, 10-Internal carotid artery, 11-Tuberculum sellae, 12-Sinus intercavernous, 13-Sinus cavernous, 14-Diaphragma sellae, 15-Sinus intercavernous, 16-Dorsum sellae, 17-Internal carotid artery, 18-Oculomotor nerve, 19-Superior petrosal sinus, 20-Abducens nerve, 21-Trigeminal nerve, 22-Trochlear nerve, 23- Ttrigeminal (semilunar)ganglion, 24-Mandibular nerve, 25 – Accessory meningeal ramus, 26-Medial meningeal artery and veins, 27-Maxillary nerve, 28-Ophthalmic nerve, 29-Ophthalmic artery, 30-Optic nerve, 31-Superior ophthalmic vein, 32-Muscular arteries, 33-Lateral rectus muscle, 34-Lacrimal artery, 35-Inferior rectus muscle, 36-Posterior ciliary artries, 37-Lacrimal vein, 38-Vorticosa vein, 39- Superior rectus muscle, 40-Lacrimal gland, 41-Episcleral veins, 42- Eyeball, 43-Superior oblique muscle, 44-Cornea, 45-Nasofrontal vein, 46-Frontal bone, 47-trochlea, 48-Supraorbital artery (Sketch is made on the base Sinelnikov R.D., Sinelnikov JA.R., Sinelnikov A.JA.: Atlas of human anatomy, Novaja volna, Moscow, 2007-2010).

1.12.1. Ophthalmic Artery

The ophthalmic artery originates from the internal carotid artery, immediately after its exit from the cavernous sinus. The artery spreads obliquely frontward and laterally, and together with the optic nerve enters the orbit through the optical canal. At the posterior part of the orbit the artery lies between the optic nerve and the abducens nerve. Going under the superior rectus muscle and the upper eyelid levator muscle, the ophthalmic artery approaches the medial orbital wall. The ophthalmic artery usually produces ten side branches, but their number considerably varies.

1. The central artery of retina. *(a. centralis retinae)* most frequently is the first side branch of the ophthalmic artery. Adherent with the lateral side of the optic nerve it is directed frontward, and then, 10-12 mm behind the sclera, it penetrates membranes of optic nerve and enters inside the nerve through its lateral and inferior surface. Following the nerve axis, the artery reaches its papilla on the retina, in which it forks into the upper and lower terminal branch. The terminal branches of the central artery of retina are most frequently the four small arteries of retina.

2. The lacrimal artery *(a. lacrimalis),* together with the central retinal artery, derives from the posterior part of the ophthalmic artery. The lacrimal artery forks into numerous branches: muscular branches, for lateral rectus muscle, zygomatic branch, which enters the zygomatic bone canal with the zygomatic nerve, lacrimal branches, for the vascularization of lacrimal gland and lateral palpebral branches, which bring the blood to the lateral ends of the upper and the lower eyelid and there anastomose with the palpebral medial arteries *(aa. palpebrales mediales)* which are direct branches of ophthalmic artery.

3. The posterior short ciliary arteries *(aa. ciliares posteriores breves)* fork into four to five short arteries. The posterior short ciliary arteries spread frontward to the posterior segment of the sclera, penetrate it around the opening of the optic nerve and enter into the perichoroid space. These arteries supply the choroid and the superficial layers of retina.

4. The posterior long ciliary arteries *(aa. ciliares posteriores longae)* pass above the optic nerve and through the sclera they reach the choroid.

5. Muscular branches *(rami musculares)* arise directly from the ophthalmic artery, or some of its side branches, and supply blood to the extraocular muscles. The upper muscular branch has a smaller caliber than the lower and gives branches for levator palpebrae superioris muscle, superior oblique muscle and medial rectus muscle. The inferior muscular branch is larger than the upper one and gives branches for inferior rectus muscle, inferior oblique muscle an lateral rectus muscle.

6. The supraorbitalis artery *(a. supraorbitalis)* derives from the ophthalmic artery at its intersection with the upper side of the optic nerve and spreads frontward along the orbital roof and above levator palpebre superior muscle, for which it provides several branches. The supraorbital artery, together with the lateral branch of the supraorbital nerve, passes through the bony supraorbital incisure, i.e., through the same-named opening and exits the orbit. Then it takes a route upwards along the forehead and forks into two or three final branches. In the orbit, the supraorbital artery supplies blood to the extrabulbar muscles and the periosteum. In the forehead, it vascularizes the frontal bone and the soft tissues of the frontal region.

7. The posterior ethmoidal artery *(a. ethmoidalis posterior)* forms at the medial side of the optic nerve and spreads medially. After passing through the posterior ethmoidal foramen, on the superior medial orbital margin, it enters the anterior cranial fossa.

8. The anterior ethmoid artery *(a. ethmoidalis anterior)* forms in front of the posterior ethmoid artery, and like the aforementioned it reaches the anterior cranial fossa through the anterior ethmoidal foramen and lands on the upper side of cribriform lamina.

9. The medial palpebral arteries *(aa. palpebrales mediales)* – the upper and the lower, derive separately or by a joint trunk, in the area of the trochlea in the superior medial corner of the orbit. The medial palpebral arteries go laterally to the corresponding eyelid where they participate in the formation of the arterial arches (*arcus palpebralis superior et inferior).*

10. The supratrochlear artery *(a. supratrochlearis*) derives from the ending of the ophthalmic artery and together with the medial branch of the supraorbital nerve it exits the orbit through the frontal incisure on the superior margin of the orbital aperture. After exiting the orbit the supratrochlear artery forks into two or three branches going upwards toward the medial frontal area and supply the bone and the soft tissues.

The terminal branch – In the area of the superior medial corner of the orbit the ophthalmic artery ends as a dorsal nasal artery *(a. dorsalis nasi).* It exits the orbit passing above medial palpebral ligament, comes under the skin of the nose root where it is connected to the artery of the ocular angle *(a. angularis),* the final branch of the facial artery. Through this anastomosis a connection between the external and the internal carotid artery is formed.

1.12.2. Infraorbital Artery

The infraorbital artery is a large side branch of the maxillary artery *(a. maxillaris)* and, directed frontwards, together with the infraorbital nerve, it enters the orbit through the inferior orbital fissure. Inside the orbit the artery is positioned in the infraorbital sulcus, and then it enters *canalis infraorbitalis* on the orbital floor.

The artery exits the infraorbital canal through infraorbital foramen, comes to the anterior side of the body of the maxilla where it forms terminal branches. The infraorbital artery forks into the orbital branches, which separate from it in the infraorbital sulcus and vascularize the inferior orbital muscles and the periosteum, and the anterior superior alveolar arteries *(aa. alveolares superiores anteriores),* which separate in the infraorbital canal and supply the frontal teeth and the mucous membrane of the maxillary sinus with blood. After exiting the infraorbital opening, the infraorbital artery gives out numerous terminal branches, which dissipate all around and carry blood to the lower eyelid, the cheek and the upper lip.

1.13. Orbital Veins

The vein blood from the orbit and its content is carried out by the superior and the inferior ophthalmic vein, which are the tributaries to the venous cavernous sinus. According to some researches, the vein blood from the orbit flows to both cavernous sinuses, and also towards the facial vein (Figures 7, 8).

The superior ophthalmic vein (*vena ophthalmica superior)* represents the main orbital vein, and it is formed in the area of the superior medial corner of the orbit, where it is connected with the angular vein *(v. angularis)* from which the facial vein *(v. facialis)* starts. This anastomosis, which may be quite large, is important in practice because through it and the superior ophthalmic vein the purulent processes from the upper lip and other areas of the face may be transmitted to the cavernous sinus and the brain membranes. On its way through the orbit the superior ophthalmic vein mainly follows the trunk of the ophthalmic artery. The vein from the superior medial corner of the orbit goes directly backwards along the superior medial orbital margin and then turns laterally and backwards intersecting the upper side of the ophthalmic artery and the optic nerve. The vein finally passes from the orbit to the middle cranial fossa through the lateral end of the superior orbital fissure, and ends by flowing into the anterior end of the cavernous sinus.

The inferior ophthalmic vein *(vena ophthalmica inferior)* is usually the main tributary of the superior ophthalmic vein and it is considerably smaller than it. It forms in the area of the inferior medial corner of the orbit and then it spreads across the orbital floor obliquely backwards and laterally, under the eyeball and the optic nerve. In the vicinity of the orbital apex the vein is positioned between inferior and lateral rectus muscles and then it flows into the superior ophthalmic vein. The inferior ophthalmic vein sometimes directly flows into the anterior end of the cavernous sinus.

1.14. Lymphatic System of the Orbit

The lymphatic system of the orbit and of the accessory organs of the eye has been well developed. The lymphatic vessels from the lateral area of the orbit, the eyelids, the conjunctiva and the lacrimal glands spread laterally and flow into the parotid lymph nodes (*nodi lymphatici parotidei*). The lymphatic vessels from the medial area of the orbit, the eyelids, the conjunctiva, the lacrimal sac and the nasolacrimal duct mostly follow the angular vein and the facial vein and flow into the submandibular lymph nodes (*nodi lymphatici submandibulares*).

1.15. Orbital Nerves

The innervation of the eye and its accessory organs is achieved through six peripheral cerebral nerves whose functions are quite different. Those are: optic nerve, oculomotor nerve, trochlear nerve, trigeminal nerve, abducens nerve, and facial nerve (Figures 7, 9, 10).

1.15.1. Optic Nerve (N. Opticus)

The optic nerve ostensibly starts from the anterior lateral angle of the optic chiasm *(chiasma opticum),* where the fibers of the right and the left optic nerve intersect partially. From optic chiasm the nerve mainly spreads frontward and laterally, and it is positioned in the middle cranial fossa, then passes through the bony optic canal *(canalis opticus),* entering the orbit. The optic nerve then, winding through the orbit, enters the eyeball, 4 mm medially and around 1 mm below the posterior pole of the eyeball. The winding direction of the optic nerve allows smooth movements of the eyeball, without stretching the nerve. In the horizontal plane the optic nerve has the shape of the letter S. With some patients, for example, suffering from the orbital tissue oedema and exophthalmos, with protruded eyeball, there are no significant visual obstructions due to the winding direction of the optic nerve. The total nerve length is about 50 mm. In the optic canal the nerve trunk has the same length as the canal, 8-10mm, and spreads frontwards, laterally and downwards.

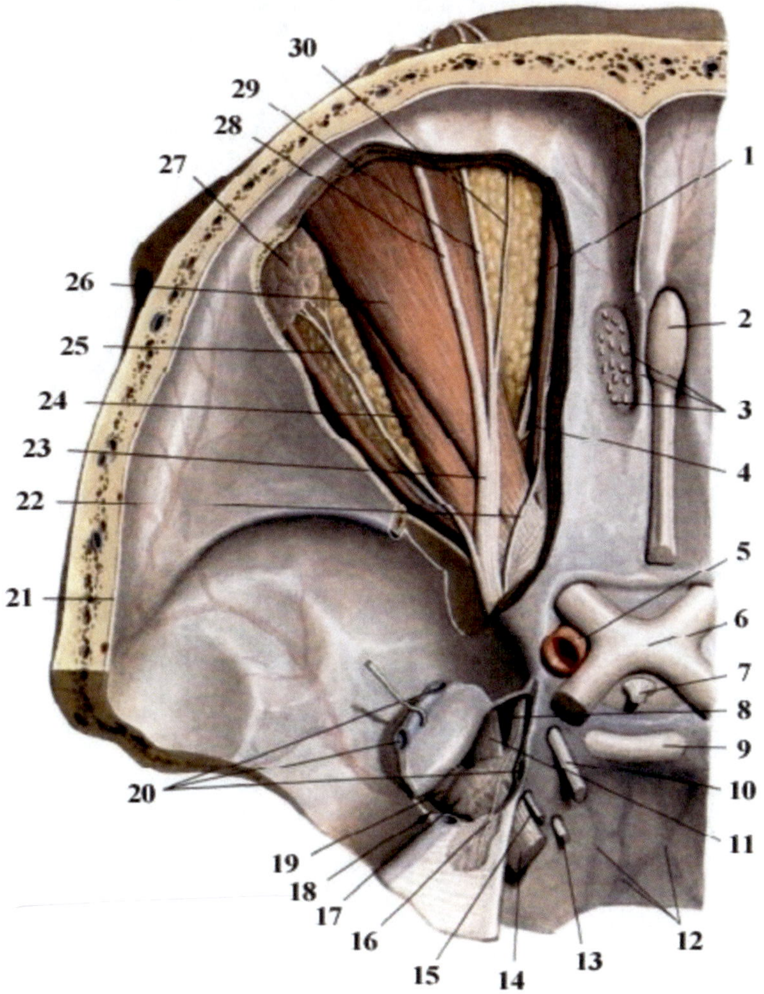

Figure 9. Orbital nerves - higher horizontal cross section. 1- Superior oblique muscle, 2.- Olfactory bulb, 3 - Olfactory nerves, 4 - Nasociliary nerve, 5 - Internal carotid artery, 6 - Optic chiasm, 7 - Infundibulum, 8 - Ophthalmic nerve, 9 - Dorsum sellae, 10 - Oculomotor nerve, 11 - maxillary nerve, 12 - Basilar plexus, 13 - Trochlear nerve. 14 -Trigeminal nerve, 15 - Abucens nerve, 16 - Ramus tentorii, 17 - Trigeminal ganglion, 18 - Trigeminal cavum, 19 - Mandibular nerve, 20 - Superior petrosal sinus, 21 - Dura mater, 22 - Trochlear nerve, 23 - Frontal nerve, 24 - Superior rectus muscle, 25 - Lacrimal nerve, 26 - Levator palpebre muscle, 27 - Lacrimal gland, 28 - Supraorbital nerve – lateral branch, 29 - Supraorbital nerve – medial branch, 30 - Supratrochlear nerve (Sketch is made on the base Sinelnikov R. D., Sinelnikov JA. R., Sinelnikov A. JA.: Atlas of human anatomy, Novaja volna, Moscow, 2007-2010).

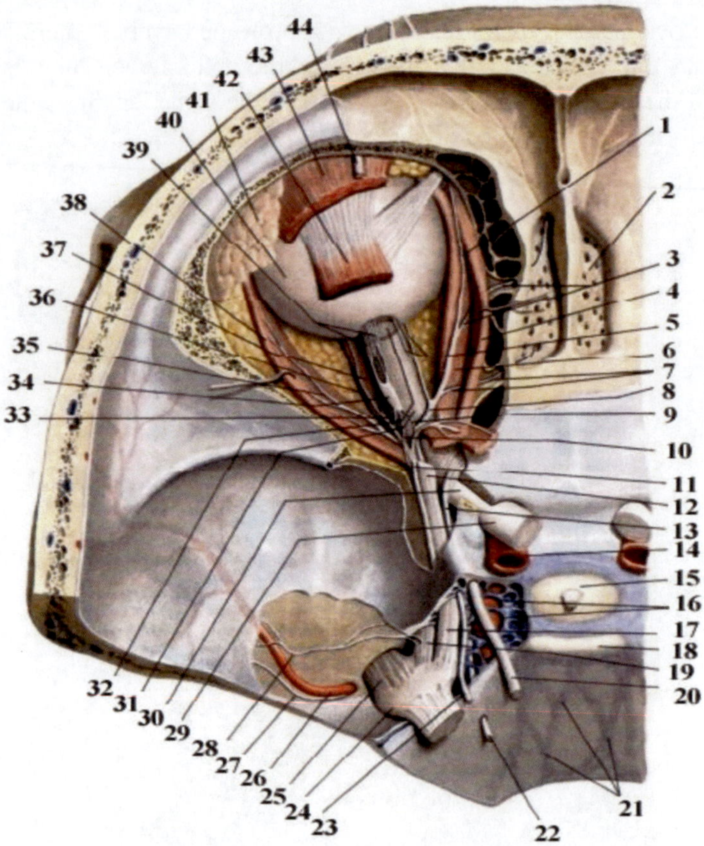

Figure 10. Orbital nerves – lower horizontal cross section. 1 – Infratrochlear nerve, 2 – Cribriform plate, 3 – Anterior ethmoidal nerve, 4 – Superior oblique muscle, 5 – Long ciliary nerves, 6 – Medial rectus muscle, 7 – Posterior ethmoidal nerve, 8 – Accessory nerve, 9 – Communicating branch with the ciliary ganglion, 10- Sympathetic root to the ciliary ganglion, 11 – Lacrimal nerve, 12 – Frontal nerve, 13 –Trochlear nerve, 14 – Internal carotid artery, 15 – Hypophysis, 16 – Cavernous plexus, 17 – Ophthalmic nerve, 18 – Dorsum selae, 19 – Maxillary nerve, 20 – Oculomotor nerve, 21 – Basilar plexus, 22 – Abducens nerve, 23 -Trochlear nerve, 24 – Trigeminal ganglion, 25 – Mandibular nerve, 26 – Medial meningeal artery, 27 – Meningeal branch of mandibular nerve, 28 – Medial meningeal branch, 29 – Optic nerve – intracranial part, 30 – Optic nerve – intracanalicular part, 31 – Optic nerve – orbital part, 32 – Optic nerve – intraocular part, 33 – Parasympathetic root from oculomotor nerve, 34 – Ciliary ganglion, 35 – Abducens nerve, 36 – Inferior division of oculomotor nerve, 37 – Inferiir rectus muscle, 38 – Lateral rectus muscle, 39 – Short ciliary nerves, 40 – Eye bulb, 41 – Lacrimal gland, 42 – Superior rectus muscle, 43 – Levator palpebrae superioris muscle, 44 – Supraorbital nerve (Sketch is made on the base Sinelnikov R. D., Sinelnikov JA. R., Sinelnikov A. JA.: Atlas of human anatomy, Novaja volna, Moscow, 2007-2010).

Together with the nerve the ophthalmic artery also passes through the canal. It is beneath the nerve and slightly laterally, penetrates its dural membrane *(vagina externa n. optici).*

In the optic canal the nerve is closely related to the sphenoid sinus and the posterior ethmoid cells, and in exceptional cases with the frontal sinus. The optic canal is in most of the cases in relation with the sphenoid sinus cavity only through the inferior wall, which is narrow and usually very thick.

In the orbit the optic nerve is around 30 mm long and it enters through the tendon annulus of Zinn medially from the oculomotor and the nasociliary nerve. The optic nerve then passes through the axis of the muscular cone formed out of the rectus extrabulbar muscles, and further goes winding through the retrobulbar fat tissue.

In the eyeball the optic nerve is about 0.6 – 0.7 mm long which corresponds to the thickness of the sclera and the choroid, and it gradually narrows passing through the openings on those membranes, so the nerve diameter of 3 mm decreases in the intrabulbar segment to 1.5 mm.

1.15.2. Oculomotor Nerve (N. Oculomotorius)

The oculomotor nerve passes through the internal wider segment of superior orbital fissure, i.e., through annulus of Zinn and enters the orbit. Already while passing through the superior orbital fissure the nerve forks into the superior and the inferior terminal branch. In the orbit the terminal branches of the oculomotor nerve diverge. The superior branch *(ramus superior)* gives a lateral branchlet for superior rectus muscle and a medial branchlet for levator palpebrae superioris muscle. The inferior branch *(ramus inferior)* is of a much larger caliber than the superior one and spreads frontwards under the optic nerve then forking into three branchlets: medial – for medial rectus muscle, central – for inferior rectus muscle, and lateral – for inferior obliquus muscle. The long path of the oculomotor nerve and its close relations with the bone explain the frequent injuries of this nerve.

1.15.3. Trochlear Nerve (N. Trochlearis)

The trochlear nerve is exclusively a motor nerve that innervates the superior oblique muscle. Trochlear nerve is the thinnest brain nerve, but with a longest path through the cranial cavity. It enters the orbit through the superior orbital fissure, running obliquely frontwards and medially, directly under the orbital roof, and with 3-4 branches it enters the superior oblique muscle.

1.15.4. Three-Branched or Trigeminal Nerve (N. Trigeminus)

The trigeminal nerve coming out of the brain at the border between the anterior (ventral) and a corresponding lateral side of the pons, with two roots – the motor one (*radix motoria)* and the sensitive (*radix sensoria).* The sensitive root is of a much larger caliber with the added sensitive trigeminal Gasser's ganglion. Three final branches of the nerve exit from the anterior convex margin of the ganglion: ophthalmic nerve, maxillary nerve an mandibular nerve.

1.15.5. Ophthalmic Nerve (N. Ophthalmicus)

The ophthalmic nerve exits from the anterior convex margin of the trigeminal ganglion and it is directed frontwards and slightly upwards, and passes between the two leaves of the dura mater which form the lateral wall of the cavernous sinus. Trochlear nerve is positioned above the ophthalmic nerve, and maxillar nerve is placed under it and laterally. Directly behind the superior orbital fissure or, sometimes, when passing through the fissure, the ophthalmic nerve forks into three terminal branches: lacrimal nerve *(n. lacrimalis)*, frontal nerve *(n. frontalis)* and nasociliary nerve *(n. nasociliaris)*.

The lacrimal nerve is the lateral and the thinnest terminal branch of the ophthalmic nerve. Immediately behind the lacrimal gland the lacrimal nerve gives out the anastomatic branch with the zygomatic nerve *(r. anastomoticus cum n. zygomatico)*. By this anastomosis the parasympathetic fibers of the facial nerve join inside the lacrimal nerve.

The frontal nerve is the central and the largest terminal branch of the ophthalmic nerve. The frontal nerve passes through the superior orbital fissure laterally from the annulus of Zinn and trochlear nerve, and medially from the lacrimal nerve. In the orbit, the frontal nerve is directed frontwards, directly under the orbital roof and above levator palpebrae superioris musle. In the area of the orbital apex the frontal nerve intersects the upper side of the trochlear nerve which spreads obliquely towards the middle. At a various distance from the superior margin of the orbital aperture, in most cases 4-5 mm behind this margin, frontal nerve gives out its terminal branches - supraorbital and supratrochlear nerve.

The nasociliary nerve is the terminal branch of the ophthalmic nerve, which enters the orbit through the annulus of Zinn, medially from the terminal branches of the oculomotor nerve. Inside the orbit the nerve spreads obliquely frontwards and medially. Through the fat tissue, between the optic nerve and medial rectus muscle, following the trunk of the ophthalmic artery, it reaches the anterior ethmoid opening where it forks into two final branches. On the way through the orbit nasociliary nerve produces three side branches. The anastomotic branch for the ciliary ganglion *(r. communicans cum ganglione ciliari)* detaches from the nasociliary nerve immediately upon its entering the orbit. It follows the lateral side of the optic nerve, and then reaches the ciliary ganglion in which it also ends. The long ciliary nerves *(nn. ciliares longi)*, which usually come in pairs, separate from the nasociliary nerve above the upper side of the optic nerve. Spreading frontwards, following the medial side of the optic nerve, they finally penetrate the sclera together with the short ciliary nerves and enter the eyeball. The long ciliary nerves innervate the eyeball membranes by sensitive fibers, and dilatator pupillae muscle by sympathetic fibers. The sympathetic fibers come from the sympathetic internal carotid plexus (*plexus caroticus internus)* and its anastomosis with the ophthalmic nerve trunk. The posterior ethmoidal nerve *(n. ethmoidalis posterior)* spreads medially and, after passing through the eponymous opening, enters the anterior cranial fossa, and then reaches the roof of the nasal cavity through the openings at the back end of cribriform plate. In the area of the anterior ethmoidal opening the nasociliary nerve forks into two final branches. The anterior ethmoidal nerve *(n. ethmoidalis anterior)* spreads medially and through the same-named opening passes from the orbit to the anterior cranial fossa and then through the opening at the anterior end of cribriform plate it reaches the anterior part of the nasal cavity roof where it finally ends. The infratrochlear nerve *(n. infratrochlearis)* spreads frontwards, continues in the direction of the nasociliary nerve, and under the trochlea it reaches the superior medial corner of the orbit where it gives branches for the upper and the lower eyelid, lacrimal sac and the nose root skin.

The ciliary ganglion (*ganglion ciliare)* belongs to an autonomous nervous system and is added to the ophthalmic nerve. The size of the ciliary ganglion varies from 1x1mm to 3x4 mm. It has the shape of a rectangular grayish plate, lying inside the orbit on the lateral side of the optic nerve. Ciliary ganglion, like other autonomous ganglions, has afferent, preganglionic and efferent, postganglionic fibers (sensitive, parasympathetic and sympathetic).

1.15.6. Maxillary Nerve (N. Maxillaris)

The maxillary nerve is only a sensitive nerve, but some of its side branches are also joined by the parasympathetic fibers, which reach the lacrimal gland, the palatal and nasal glands through the pterygopalatine ganglion. The maxillary nerve innervates the middle part of the dura mater, skin of the central facial area and the lower eyelid, the mucous membrane of the nasal cavity, the upper lip, the hard and the soft palate, the teeth and gums of the maxilla. The terminal branch of the maxillary nerve i.e., infraorbital nerve (*n. infraorbitalis)* and pteriogopalatine ganglion, which is added to the maxillary nerve trunk, innervates the orbital region. The maxillary nerve gives out the largest number of side branches in the pterygopalatine fossa. Among them the following four are the most important ones: zigomatic nerve *(n. zygomaticus),* pterygopalatine nerves *(nn. pterygopalatini),* posterior superior alveolar branches *(rr.alveolares superiors posteriores)* and infraorbital nerve *(n. infraorbitalis).* Zigomatic nerve, passing through the inferior orbital fissure on the lateral wall of the orbit, anastomoses with the lacrimal nerve by a communication branch *(r. communicans cum n. zygomatico),* and then it enters the bony canal of the zygomatic bone. Pterygopalatine nerves, 2-3 of them in most of the cases, represent short afferent and efferent branches of the pterygopalatine ganglion. The posterior superior alveolar branches, which are connected with other alveolar branches, form the superior dental plexus *(plexus dentalis superior).* The infraorbital nerve passes across the floor of the orbit and therefore will be described in more detail.

The infraorbital nerve is the largest and terminal branch of the maxillary nerve. After passing through the inferior orbital fissure, the infraorbital nerve enters infraorbital sulcus at the orbital floor, and then dives into the infraorbital canal. It exits this canal through the infraorbital opening on the anterior side of the maxilla. When passing through the infraorbital sulcus and the canal the infraorbital nerve comes to a close relation with the maxillary sinus cavity, from which it is separated by a thin paper-like bony wall, which is sometimes even dehiscent. In the infraorbital sulcus and canal the infraorbital nerve forks into alveolar branches. After exiting the infraorbital opening on the anterior side of the maxilla it then forks into numerous final branches: inferior palpebral branches *(rr. palpebrales inferiores),* external nasal branches *(rr. nasales externi),* internal nasal branches (*rr. nasales interni)* and upper labial branches *(rr. labiales superiores).*

The pterygopalatine ganglion *(ganglion pterygopalatinum)* has been added to the maxillary nerve trunk and it is located in the pterygopalatine fossa, inserted into the anterior opening of the pterygoid canal *(canalis pterygoideus).* The afferent preganglionic fibers of the pterygopalatine ganglion are: pterygopapalatine nerves *(nn. ptreygopalatini),* major petrosal nerve *(n. petrosus major)* and deep petrosal nerve *(n. petrosus profundus).* Pterygopalatine nerves bring sensitive fibers from the maxillary nerve to the ganglion, but also dispatches the fibers from the ganglion.

The major petrosal nerve represents the parasympathetic branch of the facial nerve. The deep petrosal nerve brings the sympathetic fibers to the ganglion. The efferent postganglionic fibers of the pterygopalatine ganglion join the short pterygopalatine nerves. Through them they go to the zygomatic nerve for the innervation of the lacrimal gland by the anastomosis with the lacrimal nerve *(r. communicans cum n. zygomatic).* The mentioned postganglionic fibers also go to the terminal nerve branches which innervate nasal and palatal glands.

1.15.7. Abducens Nerve (N. Abducens)

The abducens nerve is exclusively a motor nerve that innervates lateral rectus muscle. After exiting the anterior end of the cavernous sinus, abducens nerve passes through the annulus of Zinn and enters the orbit. Inside the orbit abducens nerve leans against the deep side of the lateral rectus muscle and then it forks into 4-5 branches and penetrates this muscle.

1.15.8. Facial Nerve (N. Facialis)

The facial nerve is a mixed brain nerve which, apart from the motor and sensitive ones, also contains the parasympathetic fibers. The motor fibers of the facial nerve innervate the striated subcutaneous muscles of the head, the platysma, the stylochiloid muscle, the posterior belly of the digastric muscle and stapedius muscle. The sensitive fibers are the part of the intermedius nerve and contain afferent, gustoreceptory fibers, which come from the fungiform papillae on the tongue. The parasympathetic fibers of the facial nerve are the efferent secretory fibers, which go through the major petrosal nerve into the pterygopalatine ganglion, and then into the lacrimal gland, the nasal glands and the salivary glands of the palate. Also these fibers, through the tympanic cord *(chorda tympani)* and the lingual nerve *(n. linqualis),* go into the submandibular ganglion and then into the submandibular salivary gland. The facial nerve enters the parotid gland through the stylomastoid foramen *(foramen stylomastoideum)* where it forks into two short final trunks – the superior and the inferior, which then fork manifoldly and anastomose forming the parotid plexus *(plexus parotideus)* in the parotid gland. The final branches of this plexus - *rr. temporales, rr. zygomatici, rr. bucales, r. marginalis mandibulae* and *r. colli* innervate the subcutaneous head muscles and the platysma.

1.16. Orbital Fat Body (Corpus Adiposum Orbitae)

The fat tissue of the orbit fills the orbit between its walls, the eyeball and its accessory organs. This tissue is unequally developed. In thin persons it is scarce, so the eyeballs are pulled in, while in obese people it is vice versa. The fat tissue has both mechanical and protective function and adjusts to the movements of the eyeball, the muscle and the eyelids. The retrobulbar and the parabulbar part of the orbital fat tissue can be differentiated.

The retrobulbar part fills the retrobulbar space. The fat tissue there is limited by the peripheral muscular cone formed by the extraocular rectus muscles. The connective extensions spreading from the deep sides of the rectus muscles fascias and from the posterior side of Tenon's capsule divide this fat tissue in the lobules. The optic nerve winds through the central part of the fat tissue.

The parabulbar part fills the remaining part of the orbit, i.e., space between the periorbit and the muscular fasciae, and then it is extended frontward, around Tenon's capsule, to lacrimal gland and the orbital septum.

References

[1] Jovanović S., Keros P., Cvetković D., Jeličić N., Vinter I., Eye Cavity and the Organ of Vision, *Scientific Book*, Belgrade, 1989.

[2] Koornneef L., Orbital septa: anatomy and function, *Ophthalmology* 86:876, 1979.

[3] Netter F. H., Atlas of human anatomy, Ciba – Giegy Corporation, New Jersey, 1989.

[4] Sinelnikov R.D., Sinelnikov JA. R., Sinelnikov A. JA.: Atlas of human anatomy, Novaja volna, Moscow, 2007-2010.

[5] Zide B. M., Jelks G. W., *Surgical anatomy of the orbit*, Raven Press, New York, 1985.

Chapter 2

Treatment of the Orbital Fractures

2.1. Introduction

Traumatic fractures of the orbit are relatively common injuries in both wartime and peacetime. They comprise approximately 10% of head injuries [4]. These injuries occur most frequently to the face and skull, but also occur as isolated injuries.

Taking into account the specific anatomic structure, delicate position, and contents of the orbit, even today there are different opinions concerning the mechanism of occurrence and treatment of these injuries. As for surgical treatment, until recently the orbit has been a relative mystery; that is to say, no surgical discipline has classified the orbit in its domain. However, as of late, there have been an increasing number of surgeons in the craniofacial field who have mastered complete orbital surgery and orbital trauma as well.

2.2 Cause and Mechanism of Orbital Fractures

War injuries, caused by both firearms and explosives, are usually very severe and include fracture, dislocation, or destruction of the orbital walls, with injury to the orbital contents and varying degrees of damage to the eyelids. Of course, explosive injuries are also frequently associated with extensive injuries to the upper and medial thirds of the face, including brain injury. The extent and severity of wartime injuries depends on the mass and the kinetic energy of a projectile. Bearing in mind that the orbit is situated between the paranasal sinuses and the nasal cavity, blast effects also may have a role in orbital trauma.

Peacetime orbital injuries occur most frequently in traffic accidents, fights, falls on the face, and while participating in sporting events. Traffic injuries are most frequently more severe compared with other injuries. They can also be isolated or encompass the face and skull (most often they include the zygomaticomaxillary complex). Bone fractures can be linear, with smaller or larger dislocations, comminutive, or with defects. They are purely mechanical injuries. The severity of the injury depends on the force and direction of impact as well as the surface under effect of the mechanical force.

A special type of these injuries is the so-called *blowout fractures* of the orbit. The mechanism of occurrence of these injuries can be when a hard object hits the orbit (e.g., when the head is hit during a traffic accident, when the orbit receives a punch or a kick, when a ball is thrown at the orbit, etc.). The orbital contents are pushed back toward the orbital apex, into the narrower part of the orbit. The increased intraorbital pressure (hydraulic pressure) causes a break or a blowout fracture of the weakest part of the orbital wall without fracturing the orbital rim [2, 3, 4, 5, 42].

Reny and Striker [30] as well as Fujino and Makino [9] consider that a sufficiently hard impact of an object over the orbit transmits the energy to the orbital floor and causes it to collapse. Experiments [4. 9] have suggested that these injuries may be caused by both mechanisms. On impact of a hard object over the orbit, most probably both mechanisms are engaged simultaneously. These are "pure" blowout fractures. Pure blowout fractures occur most frequently from blows of the fist. If, under the effect of force, the orbital wall and the orbital rim are fractured too, then these are "impure" blowout fractures. They are mostly caused by traffic accidents. Although blowout fractures affect the orbital floor most commonly, the other walls of the orbit (especially the medial one) can be fractured by the same mechanism [4, 7, 11, 40].

Frequently, the term *blowout fracture* is used for all fractures of the orbital floor. This is a mistake. The term *blowout fracture* refers only to the mechanism of fracture occurrence.

Exceptionally rare, another mechanism can be one that is opposite to blowout—that is, blowin — which causes the so-called *blowin fractures* of the orbital walls [4, 7] with penetration of bone fragments into the orbit. This causes reduction of the orbital volume with exophthalmos as a result.

2.3. Clinical Presentation and Diagnosis

Clinical presentation and diagnosis depend on the cause, mechanism, type, and extent of injury. Severe injuries of the upper and middle third of the face with injury of the orbit are very impressive, sometimes life- threatening, with compromised breathing, abundant bleeding, liquorrhea, and a critical general state. In such patients vital functions should be managed first. As a consequence, injuries of the orbit and its contents are often neglected, and correct diagnosis is established later. The face, orbital region, eyelids, and conjunctiva are most often associated with severe edema and hematoma, which mask the injuries of the orbit and the orbital contents.

The accurate diagnosis of these injuries is complex and requires an experienced examiner. Visual inspection and palpation can provide useful data and enable timely information regarding the type and severity of the injuries. Presence of "black eye" predicts the existence of orbital fractures. In the patient in whom the eyelids can be opened, it is relatively easy to observe the position and size of the eye. In patients with more severe injuries, with a large dislocation of bone fragments, most often the eye is displaced downward and inward. Depending on the type of injury, the eye is only displaced and sometimes it is only retracted (i.e., it is "small"). If the eye is "small" orientation should be judged whether enophthalmos or bulbus perforation is in question. If the patient is conscious and can move his eyes in all directions, it is easy to notice the restricted movements of the eyeball and to hear from the patient whether he can see or whether he is seeing double images. By palpating the facial bones and the orbital rim, fracture sites (the edges of the fractured fragments, the orientation of the fracture, and the dislocation of the bone fragments) can be identified relatively easily. With a relatively quick and complete ophthalmological examination, orientation of the injuries and eye function can be assessed. The correct diagnosis of the fracture (site, type, extent, fragment dislocation) is established on the basis of radiographs of the paranasal sinuses (Waters projection), tomography of the paranasal sinuses, computed tomography (CT) of the orbit in two dimensions, three- dimensional CT, or nuclear magnetic resonance (NMR) imaging. However, most frequently, good fracture orientation is provided by plain radiographs. It is easy to observe fractures and dislocation of the orbital rim as well as fragments of the orbital floor or roof in the maxillary sinus or in the orbit. Even a fracture of the medial wall of the orbit, although it is lamina papyracea, is often seen on radiographs. If the anterior wall of the maxillary sinus is fractured and depressed under the orbital floor, usually plain radiographs present a picture of the orbital floor fracture. On CT of the paranasal sinuses, prolapse of the orbital contents toward the maxillary sinus is seen easily. Of course, CT and NMR provide precise data regarding the type and extent of the fracture as well as information about the bone defect and condition of orbital contents. The most precise data are obtained by three- dimensional CT.

The primary signs of complications due to orbital fractures are bulbus displacement, enophthalmos, diplopia, numbness of the infraorbital region, displacement of the medial and lateral canthus, ptosis or pseudoptosis of the upper eyelid, vertical shortening and eversion of the lower eyelid, various damage to the lacrimal apparatus and other accessory eye organs, different bulbus damage, and blindness.

2.3.1. Bulbus Displacement

Displacement depends on the bone fragments and ligament system dislocations [11, 15, 16, 19, 21, 26, 45]. Most commonly the zygomaticomaxillary complex is fractured with downward and backward dislocation. Together with bone structures, the periorbital and ligamentous systems are displaced as well. These cause the eye to be, to a greater or lesser degree, displaced downward and backward. Such eye displacement has enophthalmos as its sequela, whereas the upper part of the orbit is empty and is easily visible but only after resolution of eyelid edema. Due to such a dislocation of the bone fragments the longitudinal diameter of the orbit is shortened so enophthalmos is somewhat masked, it is less evident compared with its real state. If the infraorbital rim is fractured and dislocated backward, there is vertical shortening of the lower eyelid and eversion. In cases of more severe naso-orbital fractures, the nasal bones and frontal maxillary processes are displaced backward, the profile of the nose is more or less erased, and the medial orbital wall is fractured and displaced laterally. The consequence of this is traumatic telecanthus (increased width between the medial canthi because they are displaced laterally) or traumatic hypertelorism (increased intraorbital width). These injuries are often associated with injuries of the paranasal sinuses and the anterior part of the base of the skull with liquorrhea and other symptoms caused by these injuries. Fracture of the lateral zygomatic wall of the orbit with dislocation of the zygoma, mostly downward and backward, and displacement of the lateral and Lockwood ligaments in the same direction, lead to downward bulbus displacement with enophthalmos and emptiness in the upper part of the orbit.

2.3.2. Enophthalmos

Most frequently, enophthalmos is the most common sign and complication of an orbital fracture. The eye is retracted deeper into the orbit (the eye is "small"). If the cause of the enophthalmos is fracture and a defect of the medial orbital wall, then the eye is displaced medially as well. There are many conflicting theories about the cause and mechanism of occurrence of enophthalmos. The main causes are considered to be increased orbital volume (loss of bone support), post-traumatic atrophy of orbital fat tissues, loss of the support of the orbital ligaments, scarring of the orbital soft tissues, and neurogenic factors.

For a long period of time, post-traumatic atrophy of the orbital fat tissue has been considered to be the most important cause of post-traumatic enophthalmos. The neurogenic theory is based on the assumption that during trauma, damage of the orbital symphaticus and paralysis of the small Muller's muscle (which closes the lower orbital fissure) has effect on bulbus protrusion and simultaneous damage of the orbital sympathetic system leads also to atrophy of the orbital fat tissues.

Bite and colleagues [1] Manson and associates [19, 20, 21] and Roncevic [37, 38, 39] have proposed a definitive explanation of the cause and mechanism of occurrence of post-traumatic enophthalmos. The shape of the normal orbit is conical (i.e., pyramidal). The bulbar part of the orbital floor is more or less concave whereas the retrobulbar part of the orbital floor is mildly convex (Figure 1A). In cases of orbital floor fracture (or any of the orbital walls), the orbital wall is displaced outward (toward the sinuses). The orbital contents lose the support of bone and ligaments, are displaced, and take on a spherical shape (Figure 1B). The spherical shape has a smaller volume compared with the previous one. If, together with this, the orbital volume is significantly increased, because of the bone defects on the orbital walls, then enophthalmos can develop. Therefore, displacement and change of the shape of the orbital contents, and its displacement downward and backward (or medially), are the causes of enophthalmos. Change of the orbital volume correlates with the degree of enophthalmos [20].

If only the orbital floor is fractured (or any other wall) and the periosteum and ligamentous systems are intact, then there is no enophthalmos (Figure 8). Bite and colleagues [1] and Manson and associates [19, 20, 21, 22] have proved that in patients with post-traumatic enophthalmos there is no significant atrophy of the fat tissue, which can lead to evident enophthalmos. If atrophy of the orbital fat tissue is present, it could not develop so quickly and acutely after injury to cause enophthalmos, which is usually evident immediately after injury. In patients with neglected injuries due to displacement of fat tissues, entrapment, injury, scars, and pressure caused by fragments, there is significant atrophy of the orbital fat tissues because the injuries have been in effect for a longer period of time. Injuries of the orbital contents produce scars, which cause contraction. Contraction affects the excursion of the extraocular muscles, contributing also to the formation of the spherical configuration of the orbital contents. Thus, post-traumatic scars of the orbital contents can contribute to enophthalmos [20, 21, 22, 37, 38, 39].

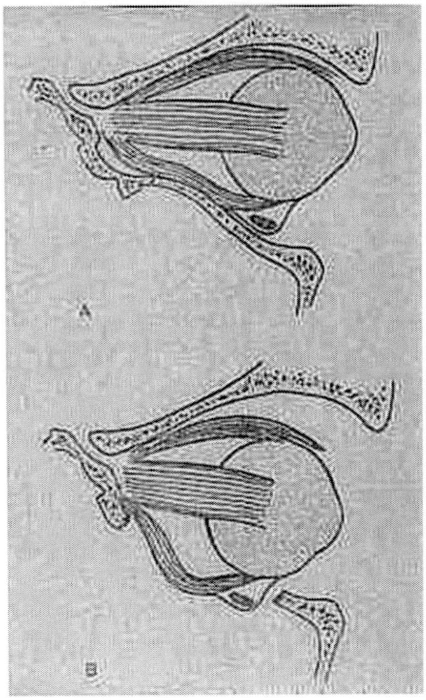

Figure 1. A- Normal shape of the orbit and normal shape and position of the orbital contents. B- After orbital floor fracture, the orbital volume is increased and the orbital contents have a spherical shape. (Reprinted with permission from Manson PN. Deep orbital reconstruction of post- traumatic enophthalmos. Clin Plast Surg 14:113-121, 1987).

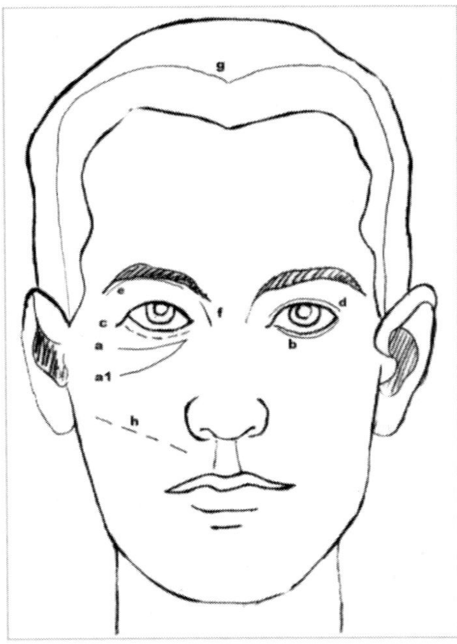

Figure 2. Surgical approach to orbit: a, a1 – lower orbitopalpebral, b – subciliar, c – conjunctival, d – upper palpebral, e – supraorbital, f – medial, g – coronal, h – bucal.

It is hard to believe that eventual paralysis of the small, thin Muller's muscle can lead to enophthalmos. Marked enophthalmos leads to pseudoptosis of the upper eyelid, deepening of the supratarsal groove, or, in cases of more manifest enophthalmos, the upper part of the orbit is empty and reduces the horizontal dimension of the palpebral opening. It is possible to obtain objective measurements of the degree of enophthalmos by exophthalmometry according to Hertl.

2.3.3. Diplopia

Bulbus displacement and enophthalmos lead to deviation of the visual axis on the injured side with diplopia as the most common sequela. Of course, together with bulbus displacement and enophthalmos, the extrabulbar muscles are displaced also. Because the orbital floor is displaced most frequently, the lower oblique and the lower straight muscles, the Lockwood ligament, and the periorbital and fascial extensions are frequently displaced and entrapped. The test of duction (i.e.,, traction) can detect whether the aforementioned muscles are entrapped due to the orbital floor fracture. The test is performed in the following manner: After local anesthesia is administered, the insertion site of the lower straight muscle or the lower oblique muscle is grasped using pincers and is pulledforward. If the muscles are entrapped due to the orbital floor fracture, their movement is restricted substantially—if movement is possible at all. However, movement can be restricted due to hematoma in the orbit. Diplopia may also be caused by damages to the nerve endings of cerebral nerves III, IV, and VI innervating the extraocular muscles, as well as because of damage, edema, or hemorrhage in these muscles.

Various combinations of enophthalmos and diplopia may occur at the orbital fracture. Both diplopia and enophthalmos are present in cases when the orbital contents are entrapped in the fracture region. Diplopia without enophthalmos occurs at the linear fracture when the orbital volume is not increased, without displacement of the orbital contents, and when a portion of the orbital contents, especially muscle, is entrapped in the linear fracture. Enophthalmos without diplopia can appear in cases of comminutive fractures or defects of the floor (wall) of the orbit with displacement and prolapse of the orbital contents, but when the orbital contents, especially the extrabulbar muscles, are not entrapped. In cases of small orbital fractures or linear orbital fractures without muscle entrapment and displacement of the orbital contents, there is no diplopia or enophthalmos. Orientation of diplopia is obtained on the basis of the patient's statement and examination, and the Hess-Lancaster test.

Anesthesia or hypoesthesia of the infraorbital region is mostly associated with fractures of the infraorbital rim and orbital floor. These changes can last for a longer period of time—up to several months. If the infraorbital nerve is torn, changes are permanent. In approximately 2% to 3% of patients, post-traumatic neuralgia of the infraorbital region is persistent.

The syndrome of the orbital upper fissure develops due to a fracture in this region and damages of cerebral nerves III, IV, parts of VI, and VI. (All these nerves pass through this fissure).

Fracture and bleeding in the region of the optic canal and orbital apex due to the pressure on the optic nerve or due to its rupture may cause blindness.

In the course of orbital fracture, damage to the lacrimal apparatus and other accessory eye organs may also occur. Various bulbus damages are also possible: from corneal abrasion to blindness due to bulbus rupture or traumatic retinal detachment. In the case of more severe injuries, especially explosive injuries, loss of the eye and accessory organs can occur.

2.4. Treatment of Orbital Fractures

Even today there is disagreement concerning the treatment of orbital fractures. It is obvious that in cases of fractures without fragment dislocations, enophthalmos, and diplopia, conservative treatment only is indicated. However, in patients with marked enophthalmos and diplopia, the prevailing attitude for a long period of time has been (especially among ophthalmologists) that surgical treatment should be avoided and that only conservative treatment should be applied [5. 8, 11, 15, 17, 27, 29, 41] In 1983, Horiono [10] conducted extensive questionnaires by mail regarding the treatment of orbital fractures. He sent questionnaires to the most famous world physicians of that time who dealt with these problems. The majority of them considered that these injuries should be treated conservatively. This attitude was defended by reports that after the application of steroid therapy, disappearance of edema and hematoma of the orbital contents as well as after eye movement exercises, enophthalmos and diplopia had disappeared, mostly after 4 to 6 months. Besides, it has been cited that after surgical treatment, postoperative enophthalmos and diplopia remained in a high percentage of patients. Also, it has been reported [27] that surgical treatment is risky due to possible complications and even a high percentage of blindness. Some however, advocated the principle that after the injury it should be awaited for consolidation of the definite state and after that, by operations on the extrabulbar muscles, diplopia and enophthalmos could be significantly or completely corrected. The previously mentioned attitudes of defending and supporting conservative treatment have currently been mainly abandoned. In cases of orbital fracture with entrapment of the orbital contents and pronounced enophthalmos and diplopia, spontaneous recovery is impossible. Additional operations on the extraocular muscles provide very modest results. These patients have permanently and significantly impaired functional and aesthetic results. Surgical therapy may provide favorable results, most often excellent. Results depend mainly on the knowledge, skill, and experience of the surgeon.

When should surgical treatment be applied? When clear indications for surgical treatment are present, such as extensive fractures, orbital wall defects, dislocation of larger fragments, marked enophthalmos, and entrapped orbital contents with diplopia, surgical treatment it should not be delayed, regardless of the presence of post-traumatic edema, except in extremely pronounced edema. The faster surgical therapy is undertaken, the better the results. Therefore, the shape and the volume of the orbit should be reconstructed as soon as possible, and the orbital contents repositioned as well. This is especially important in children. All bone injuries, especially of the face, are associated with post-traumatic edema. Except in extraordinary cases, bone surgery must not be postponed because of post-traumatic edema. The same rule applies to the orbit as well. If surgery to repair orbital fractures is postponed for various reasons, it should not be postponed longer than 7 days. Waiting for several weeks or months for the spontaneous disappearance of enophthalmos and diplopia is a professional error. On the basis of clinical presentation and other examinations, an experienced surgeon should be able to discern relatively easily the possibility of spontaneous recovery of enophthalmos and diplopia. If such a condition exists, then treat it conservatively (see Figure 8).

2.4.1. Surgical Treatment

As previously mentioned, until recently the orbit has been considered a "no-man's-land," as treatment of orbital injuries has been performed sporadically by surgeons in different specialties: ophthalmologists, and specialists in plastic and maxillofacial surgery, otorhinolaryngology, and neurosurgery. Because of this, in the past, different methods of surgical treatment have been applied. The modern concept of surgical treatment and its indications was established more than 55 years ago by John Marquis Converse [2, 3, 4, 6]' specialist in plastic and craniofacial surgery. From then until now, this concept has been gradually adopted and advanced. There are still different attitudes concerning some surgical issues, especially concerning materials used in reconstruction of orbital wall defects.

Methods of surgical treatment depend mainly on the type and extent of injury as well as the time from injury to surgery [4, 13, 21, 22, 31-39]· Taking these factors into account, orbital injuries can be classified into four groups.

Group 1: fresh bone fractures of the middle or upper third of the face with fractures of the orbital bone structures.

Group 2: fresh isolated fractures of the orbital bone structures, most commonly "pure" or "impure" blowout fractures.

Group 3: neglected fractures of the middle and upper third of the face with fractures of the orbital bone structures.

Group 4: neglected isolated fractures of the orbital bone structures, most commonly "pure" or "impure" blowout fractures.

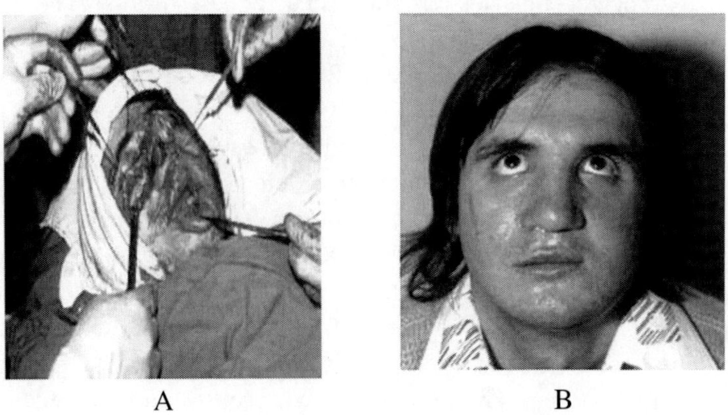

A B

Figure 3. A. Avulsion injury of the middle third of the face and nose with a defect of the zygomaticomaxillary complex and the orbital floor on the right. B. Appearance of the patient after reconstruction of the facial bone tissues and the orbit, as well as reconstruction of the soft tissues of the face and nose. Enophthalmos is corrected, no double vision, eye movements are free.

In group 1 patients (Figures 3, 4), the approach through the wounds, or in cases of closed fractures, through the lower eyelid (incision as in blepharoplasty) and the eyebrow, in combination with the approach through the mouth, or, in combination with coronary approach, that is, by an incision made at the level of the upper pole of the ear up to the opposite ear, through the hairy part of the scalp (Figure 2), it is necessary to reposition all fragments of the facial skeleton and to fix them with wire ligatures or metal mini/micro plates. To reach the orbit via the coronary incision, it is necessary to separate the scalp and periosteum from the bone, including the orbit. By repositioning the facial bones comprising the orbit, which are mostly displaced backward, the orbital volume, defects of orbital walls, and orbital diameter are increased. In this way, visible enophthalmos becomes more evident and masked enophthalmos (due to fragment dislocation and reduced orbital diameter) becomes evident. When all bone structures are repositioned, surgical treatment of the orbit is begun. By careful separation, the orbital soft tissues are freed from the fracture site, where they are trapped, or through which they have prolapsed toward the sinuses.

On freeing of the orbital contents and exploration of the rest of the orbital wall, it is necessary to avoid damaging the extrabulbar muscles, optic nerve, and infraorbital neurovascular bundle. After repositioning the orbital contents, it is necessary to reconstruct the orbital walls (i.e., the shape and volume of the orbit).

Various materials have been used to reconstruct the orbital walls (bone plates of the anterior or inner wall of the maxillary sinus, bone taken through the mouth from the chin region, iliac bone or calvaria, rib cartilage, as well as various alloplastic materials such as lyophilized bone, cartilage, and dura; and plates or nets of gold, vitallium, titanium, teflon, vicryl, platinum, proplast, silastic, hydroxylapatite, lactosorb, bioactive glass, etc. Thin alloplastic materials are generally well tolerated in the orbit and, usually, good results are achieved with these materials. However, after the use of these materials, various complications may occur, such as infection, fistulas, cysts, sinusitis, dacryocystitis, and rejection and migration of alloplastic materials, which could damage some structures of the orbital soft tissues [12, 14, 23, 24]. Of course, reconstruction with autotransplants is safer. The disadvantage of using autotransplants is that additional operations for removing autotransplants must be performed. In cases where despite good reconstruction of the shape and the volume of the orbit, enophthalmos still exists, alloplastic materials cannot be used. In these instances it is best to use a thicker part of the rib cartilage, which is shaped in the form of a wedge and positioned in such a way that the thicker part of the wedge is placed retrobulbar to the orbital apex. In this way the transplant reduces the orbital volume and pushes the bulbus forward, which leads to correction of the eye position and thus correction of the enophthalmos.

To achieve good results, regardless of the materials used for reconstruction of the orbital walls, it is necessary to separate all soft tissue of the orbit from a fracture fissure or bone defect, from the rest of the orbital wall so that material used for reconstruction is placed on the intact bone and remains at that site.

In such patients there is no need for fixation of the inserted material. If the materials used for reconstruction of the orbital wall have a good base and good support, then the orbital contents push it along the base and there is no additional dislocation. This is especially important for the most frequent fractures—orbital floor fractures. If an entire wall or the orbital rim is missing, then reconstructive materials must be fixed to the adjacent bone with wire ligatures or with metal mini/microplates. Alloplastic materials should be fixed too. After reconstruction of the medial wall and roof of the orbit, if the ethmoidal blood vessels are injured or if there is abundant bleeding, it is necessary to insert a vacuum drain into the retrobulbar space after hemostasis to prevent retrobulbar hematoma and blindness. To prevent postoperative scars around extraocular muscles, which restrict muscle function, it is necessary to begin intensive eye movement exercises on the first postoperative day.

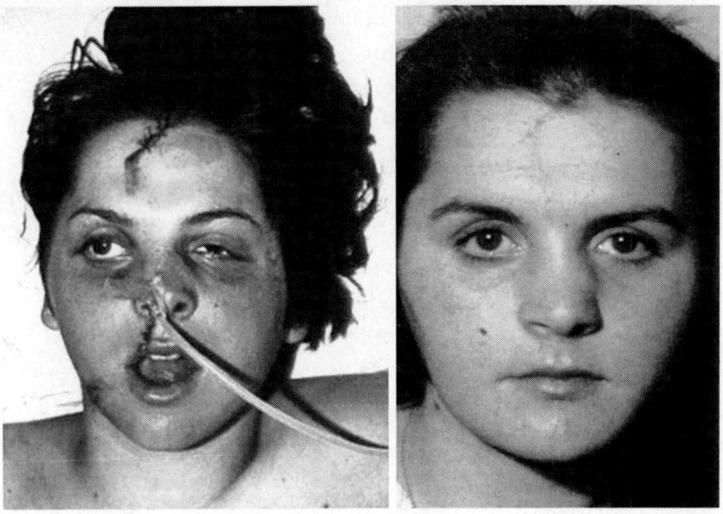

A B

Figure 4. A. Fresh fracture of the facial bones with a defect of the left orbital floor, enophthalmos, and diplopia. B. The same patient after reposition and fixation of the facial bones, and reconstruction of the left orbital floor using bone plates from the anterior wall of the maxillary sinus. Enophthalmos and double vision were corrected successfully.

In group 2 patients (Figures 5-9), the approach to the orbit, and thus the fracture site, differs. In cases of fractures of the orbital floor and infraorbital rim, the incision is placed through the lower eyelid, as in a blepharoplasty (Figure 2). The orbital wall can also be approached by an incision through the conjunctiva [43. 44]. If the lateral wall and lateral rim of the orbit are fractured, then the approach is through the lateral part of the eyebrow. If the medial orbital wall is fractured, the incision is made over the medial rim of the orbit so that the incision runs up to the level of the medial canthus. It is not placed lower, to avoid injury to the medial ligament. The orbital roof can be approached through the eyebrow and upper eyelid or transcranially. Also, the orbit can be approached via a coronary incision—an incision through the hairy part of the scalp. Of course, if several walls of the orbit are fractured, it is necessary to combine these approaches (Figure 2).

In the most common fractures—pure and impure blowout fractures—with an incision placed through the skin of the eyelid, as in a blepharoplasty (Figure 5), the skin is separated from the muscle up to the level of the infraorbital rim. At this level, the muscle is cut off and the orbit is entered at the junction of the orbital septum and periosteum by an incision through the periosteum. (The incision through the skin can be placed at a lower level; that is, at the level of the infraorbital rim. This incision is more visible later compared with the previous one.) Using a sharp raspatory, the periosteum is separated from the bone, and the entrapped orbital contents are separated from the site of entrapment or are lifted out of the sinus if they have prolapsed into it. The rest of the orbital floor is freed from the orbital contents so that the material to reconstruct the fractured orbital floor can be placed on the intact bone. For reconstruction of the orbital floor and other orbital walls, the same materials are used and in the same way as in group 1 patients. If the orbital rim is fractured at one or more sites, the fractured fragments should be repositioned previously and fixed with wire ligatures or micro/mini plates.

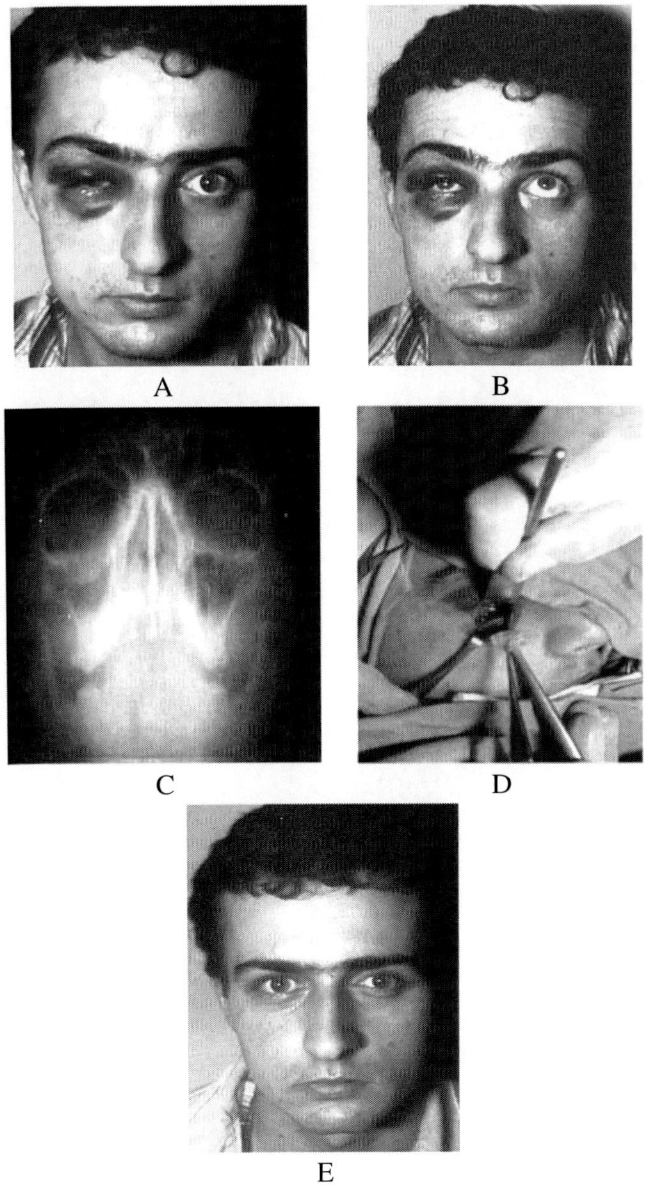

Figure 5. A. B. Fresh "pure" blowout fracture of the right orbital floor with enophthalmos, diplopia, and restricted upward eye movement. C. X-ray record. The orbital floor "hangs" in the maxillary sinus. D- Approach through the lower eyelid, the orbital floor defect is overbridged by a bone plate from the anterior wall of the maxillary sinus. E- The patient's condition after reconstruction. Enophthalmos and diplopia are corrected successfully, eye movements are free.

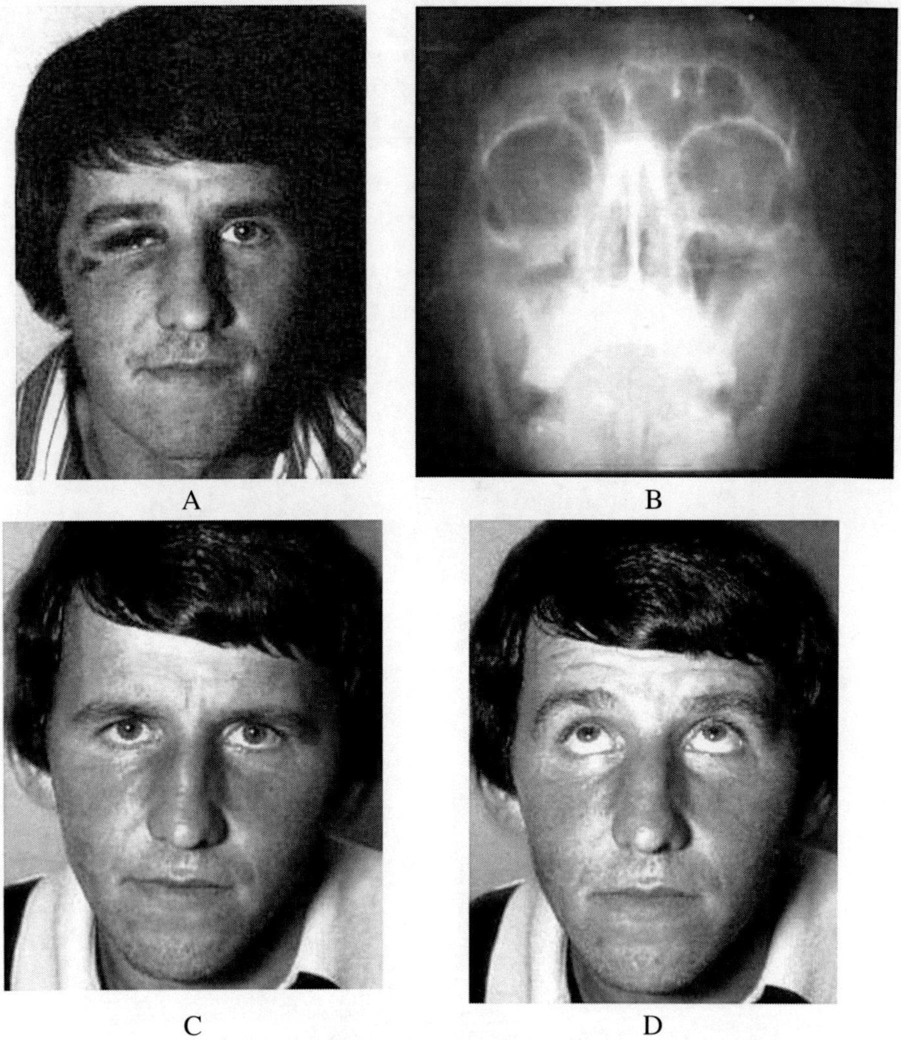

Figure 6. A, B. Fresh “pure” blowout fracture of the right orbital floor with enophthalmos, diplopia, and restricted upward eye movement). C, D. Enophthalmos and diplopia are corrected successfully, eye movements are free. Reconstruction of orbital floor is performed by a bone plate from the anterior wall of the maxillary sinus.

Injuries sustained by group 3 patients (Figures 9-12, 19, 20) are the greatest problem both for the patient and the surgeon. These are surgically neglected, or untreated or maltreated injuries with deformities of the face and orbital region, double vision, enophthalmos, hypoesthesia, anesthesia, and sometimes neuralgia of the infraorbital region as well as other defects and deformities of the accessory organs of the eye. Even today these injuries are often proclaimed to be the definite state and surgical treatment is avoided by some surgeons. In the past, deformities of the face and orbital region were corrected by using different materials (bone, cartilage, and alloplastic materials) by different approaches [18, 25] (incision over a scar; through the eyelids, eyebrows, or mouth; or by a coronary incision). Results of such operations are most commonly unsatisfactory for several reasons. It is difficult to model the contours of the face and orbital region because during the postoperative period greater or lesser resorption of the transplanted bone, displacement of alloplastic materials, or their rejection may occur. These operations cannot correct enophthalmos, diplopia, and compression of the infraorbital nerve. On the contrary, after these operations and correction of the facial contour, increase the orbital longitudinal diameter, enophthalmos becomes more evident.

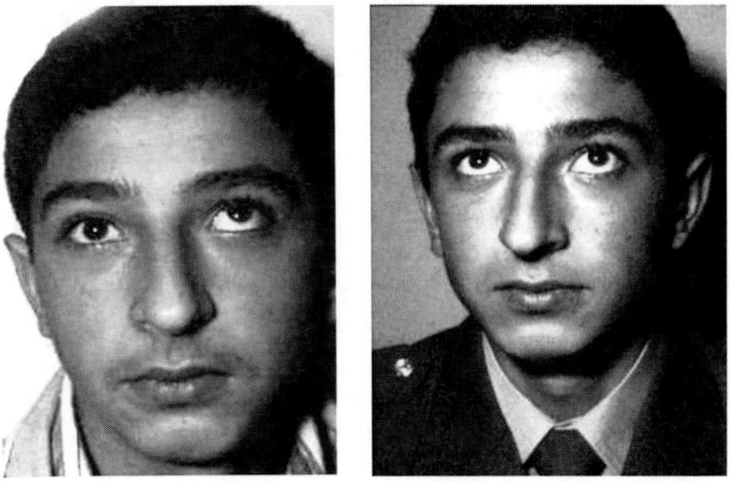

A B

Figure 7. A. Fresh "pure"blowout fracture of the right orbital floor with enophthalmos, diplopia, and restricted upward eye movement. B. Condition after reconstruction of orbital floor by a boni plate from the anterior wall of the maxillary sinus.

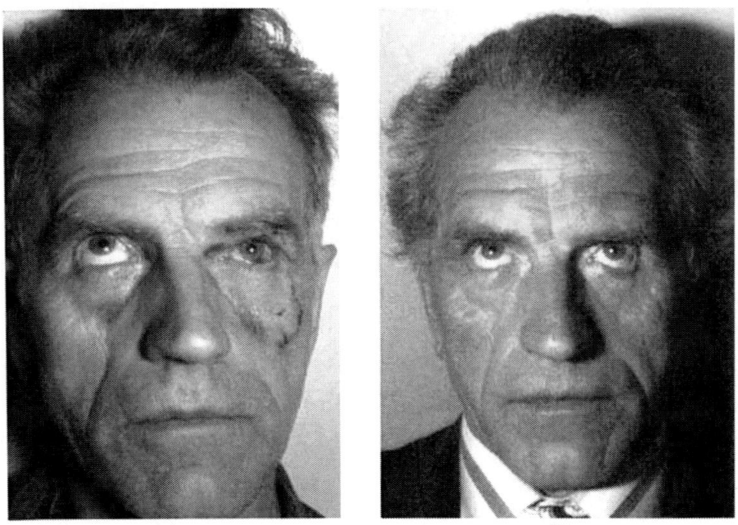

A B

Figure 8. A. "Impure" blowout fracture of the orbital floor to the left with enophthalmos, double vision, and restricted upward eye movement. B. The patient's condition after reposition and fixation of the infraorbital rim, and reconstruction of the orbital floor using iliac bone formed in the shape of a wedge. Enophthalmos and diplopia are corrected successfully, and eye movements are normal.

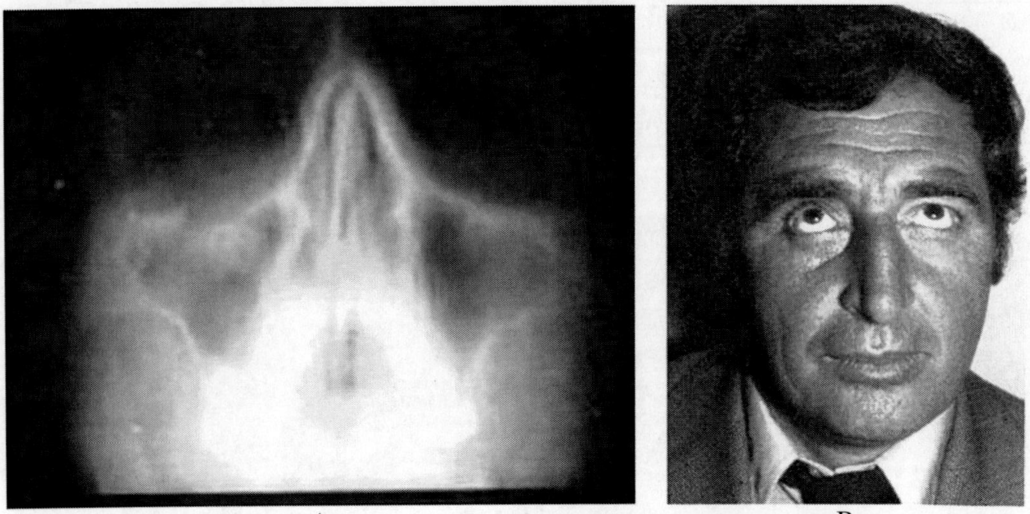

A B

Figure 9. A. Fresh "impure" blowout fracture of the orbital floor to the right. The orbital floor "hangs" in the maxillarv sinus. B. There is no enophthalmos and double vision, eye movements are free. In this case, during injuries, the orbital periosteum and ligaments system remained intact, on the anatomical position.

In such patients the method of choice is refracture; that is, osteotomy and repositioning of the fractured fragments of the facial and orbital bones [7, 33, 37, 38]· Refracture can be performed regardless of the time lapse from the injury to the surgery. Refracture is done with a osteotom and a small drill through the previous scar, eyelids, eyebrows, by approaching through the mouth and by a bicoronal, scalp approach. Usually it is necessary to combine the incision through the lateral part of the eyebrow, lower eyelid, and upper vestibulum of the oral cavity. After refracture, the fractured bone fragments can be repositioned and the contours of the face and orbital region restored completely. After repositioning, the bone fragments are fixed with wire ligatures or metal micro/mini plates. If a part of the bone is missing, it should be substituted with iliac or skull bone. If bone is used, then it is best to use the skull bone because membranous bone is less resorbed during the postoperative period compared with other bones.

Because the facial bones that support the orbital structures are most often retracted downward and backward on injury, after their refracture and reposition, the orbital diameter is increased, the defect of the orbital walls becomes larger, enophthalmos becomes more evident and masked enophthalmos evident. By repositioning the fractured fragments, the infraorbital nerve is decompressed if it has been compressed by the retracted bone fragments. Only after repositioning of the refractured fragments are the orbital contents freed from the fracture site and restored. This freeing of the orbital contents from the fracture site and their restoration is more difficult than in patients with fresh injuries due to post- traumatic scarring, which affects the orbital contents. This procedure should be performed accurately, taking care not to damage the extraocular muscles, and the infraorbital and optic nerves.

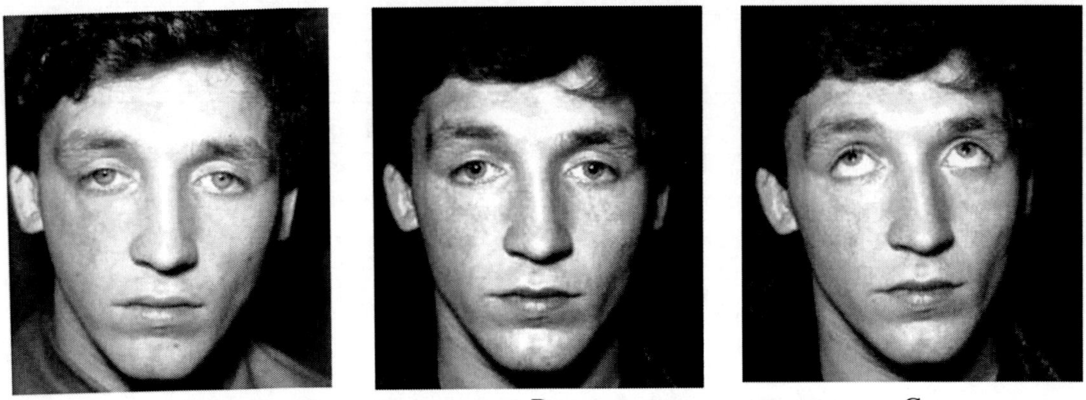

A B C

Figure 10. A. Neglected fracture of the zygomaticomaxillary complex to the right with discrete enophthalmos. The face is deformed because the zygomaticomaxillary complex is depressed backward. In this patient the longitudinal orbital diameter is shortened and enophthalmos is masked. B, C. After refracture and repositioning of the zygomaticomaxillary complex, the facial contour is restored, the orbital diameter has a normal dimension, the orbital floor defect becomes larger, and evident enophthalmos occurs. To correct the enophthalmos, the orbital floor is reconstructed using a thicker piece of rib cartilage formed in the shape of a wedge. The appearance of the face is normal, there is no enophthalmos, and eye movements are free.

After freeing and repositioning the orbital contents, this position must be preserved by reconstructing the fractured orbital walls (i.e., reconstructing the previous shape and volume of the orbit). If thin alloplastic materials are used (which is frequently done), enophthalmos and diplopia are not corrected satisfactorily even though the orbital shape and volume have been reconstructed. The orbital contents, its shape and volume, are changed definitively during a long post-traumatic period.

The evident atrophy of fat tissues occurs, and scars and contraction of the soft tissues change the shape and volume and maintain a partially spherical post-traumatic shape of the orbital contents even after their freeing from the fracture site. The spherical shape, compared with other geometric shapes, means the least volume. In a longer post-traumatic period, change of the extrabulbar muscles is evidenced too. Injuries, scars, and inactivity lead to definitive muscle changes. During the course of damage and displacement of the orbital contents and their entrapment at the fracture site, the motor nerve ends that innervate the bulbomotor muscles may also be damaged. This also can be the cause of weakened muscle function and tone, and consequently the cause of enophthalmos and diplopia, and the inability to correct completely the enophthalmos and diplopia using surgical means. All these scenarios suggest that surgical treatment of orbital injuries should not be delayed, but be done as early as possible.

In these patients it is best to use rib cartilage to reconstruct the orbital walls. It is generally not resorbed during the postoperative period. The thicker part of the cartilage should be shaped in the form of a wedge. The thicker part of the wedge is placed retrobulbarly. In this way it is possible to reconstruct the orbital shape and reduce its volume; the thicker part of the wedge placed retrobulbarly pushes the bulbus forward. Often a mistake is made by using a thicker transplant to reduce the orbital volume, which causes the eye to be lifted more vertically than necessary. Sometimes, due to post-traumatic fibrosis of the extrabulbar muscles, it is not possible to correct enophthalmos. In such cases the insertion of these muscles must be cut off.

To correct enophthalmos better, especially when the upper part of the orbit is more or less empty, it is possible (by the approach through the upper eyelid) to insert cartilage or bone into the retrobulbar space between the orbital roof and its periosteum [28, 37, 38]. However, taking into account that this transplant is placed on the periosteum, somewhat better results may not be achieved.

The first day after reconstruction of the orbit, the patient should be advised to perform eye movements in all directions to prevent postoperative scars around extraocular muscles, which can limit the function of these muscles.

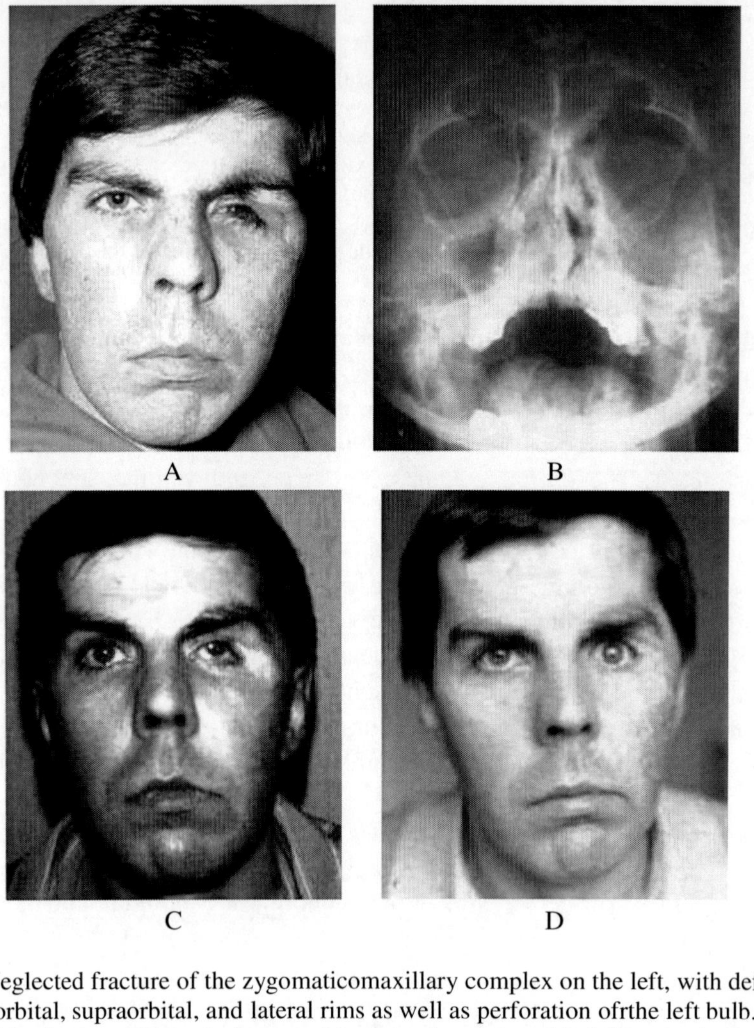

Figure 11. A. B. Neglected fracture of the zygomaticomaxillary complex on the left, with defects of the orbital floor, infraorbital, supraorbital, and lateral rims as well as perforation ofrthe left bulb. The infraorbital part of the fractured bones is depressed backward, and the orbital diameter is shortened so that enophthalmos looks less evident than it really is. C. The patient after refracture and repositioning of the fractured facial bones and after reconstruction of the orbital floor and rims using rib cartilage. Due to perforation and atrophy of the bulb and atrophy of the contents of the orbit, it is not possible to correct enophthalmos successfully. D. The patient after enucleation of the left bulbus and insertion of an eye prosthesis.

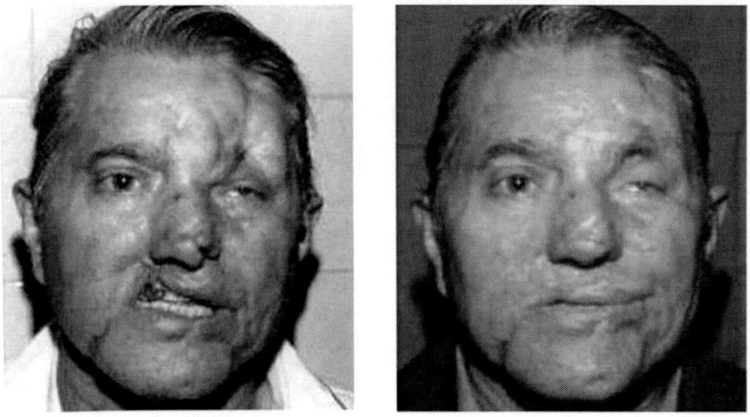

A B

Figure 12. A. Appearance of the patient 45 years after sustaining war injuries. Note the defect of the frontal, supraorbital, and infraorbital regions. Marked enophthalmos is due to perforation and atrophy of the eye, atrophy of the orbital contents and a defect of the orbital floor. There is also a post-traumatic defect of the nose and upper lip. B. After reconstruction of the frontal, supraorbital, and infraorbital regions, the longitudinal diameter of the orbit is increased and enophthalmos has become more evident. Besides reconstruction of the orbital shape and the volume of the orbit, due to marked atrophy of the eye and the orbital contents, it is impossible to correct enophthalmos. Reconstruction of the nose and the lip was performed concomitantly. The patient refused enucleation and making eye prosthesis.

In patients with extensive defects of the orbital walls and rim, it is necessary to perform a reconstruction. It is best to use rib cartilage or skull bone. If iliac bone is used, it is possible that substantial resorption may occur during the postoperative period. To reconstruct larger defects of the orbit, it is possible to transfer bone from different regions by microsurgical techniques. It is possible to transfer live, vascularized bone from the skull on the pedicle of the pericranium (i.e., on the pedicle of the superficial temporal artery and vein), (Figure 19).

In patients with orbital fracture and bulbus perforation (Figures 11, 12) despite good reconstruction of the shape and volume of the orbit, successful correction of enophthalmos is not possible because the eye is small. In such patients it is best, for several reasons, to suggest enucleation and insertion of an eye prosthesis (Figure 11).

In cases of injury of the orbit with anophthalmia, it is necessary to reconstruct the rim and walls of the orbit, the conjunctival sac, and the eyelids if they have been damaged. Only after that it is possible to construct a good prosthesis (Figures 16-20).

In group 4 patients (Figures 13, 14, 15), if impure blowout fractures are in question, refracture and reposition of the orbital rim should be performed (Figure 15). After that, as in the patients in group 3, surgical treatment of the orbit should be performed. If the orbital walls are only damaged, the approach to the walls is performed as described earlier. After dissection of the orbit, the orbital contents are freed from the fracture site and repositioned. Reconstruction of the orbital walls is performed in the same way and for the same reasons as group 3 patients.

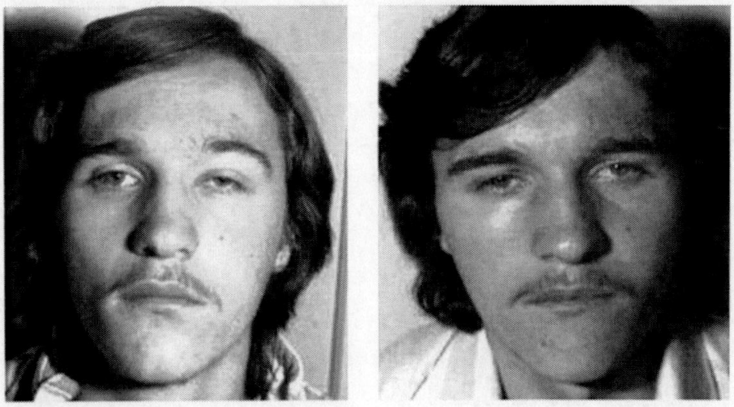

A B

Figure 13. A. Neglected "pure" blowout fracture of orbital floor with enophthalmos and diplopia. B. Condition one month after the reconstruction of the orbital floor and shape of the orbit using rib cartilage graft.

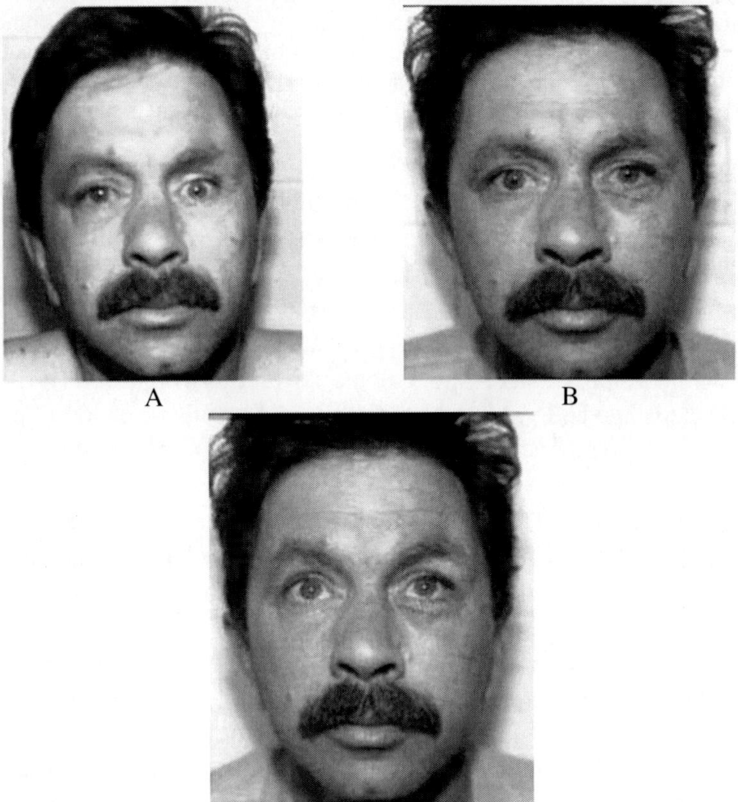

A B

C

Figure 14. A. Neglected "pure" blowout fracture of the orbital floor on the left. Upper part of the left orbit is empty. B, C. Condition seven days after reconstruction of the orbital floor and the shape by rib cartilage graft.

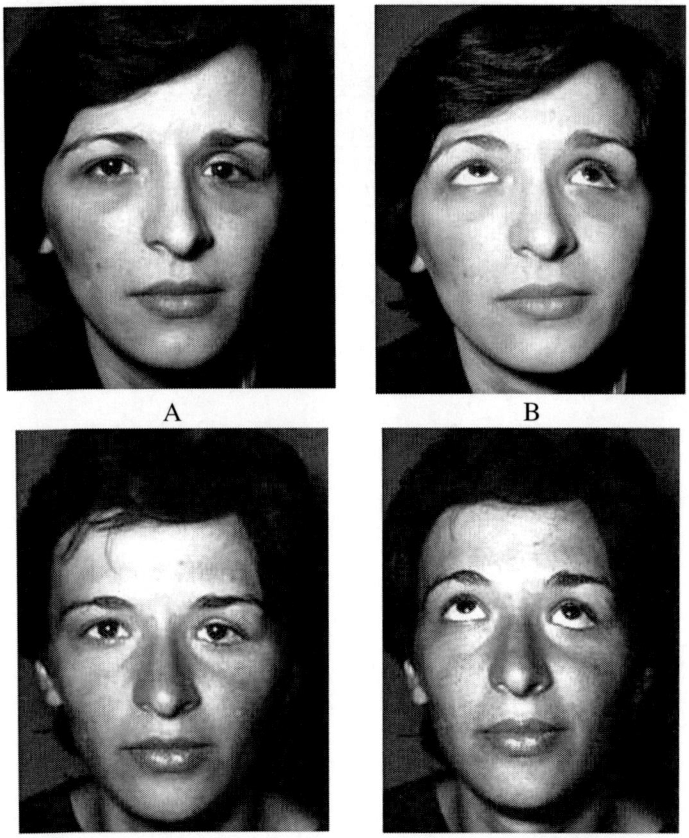

A B

C D

Figure 15. A, B. Neglected fracture of the infraorbital region and of the orbital floor on the left with enophtalmos. Upper part of the left orbit is empty. C, D. The patient after refracture and repositioning of the infraorbital region, and reconstruction of the orbital floor with an adequately formed rib cartilage graft.

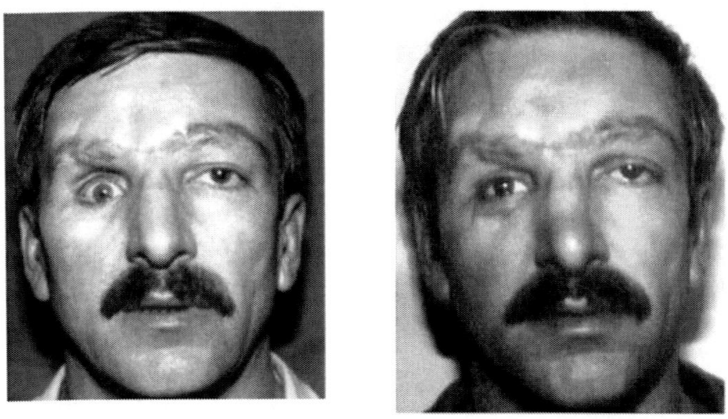

A B

Figure 16. A. Condition of the patient after injury of the right orbit with anophthalmos and eye prosthesis following 17 operations performed to provide conditions for good adaptation of the eye prosthesis. B- Condition of the patient after correction of the orbital floor, roof, and rims using rib cartilage, and correction of the conjunctival sac.

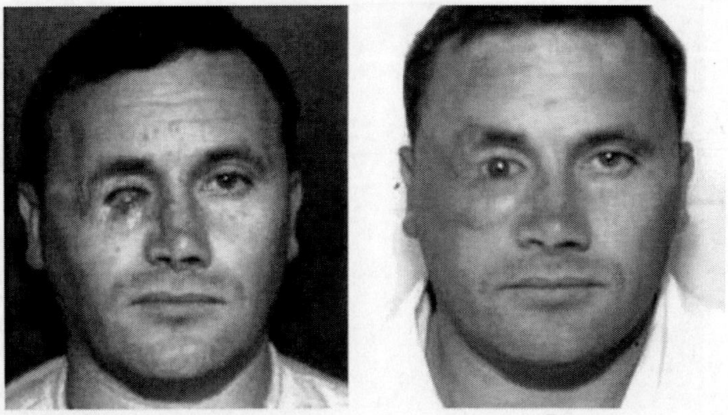

A B

Figure 17. A. Defect of the floor, lateral wall and orbital margins as well defect of eyelids and conjunctival sac with anophthalmia. B. Condition after the reconstruction of orbital walls and margins by rib carilage and reconstruction of eyelids (by forehead skin flap) and conjunctival sac.

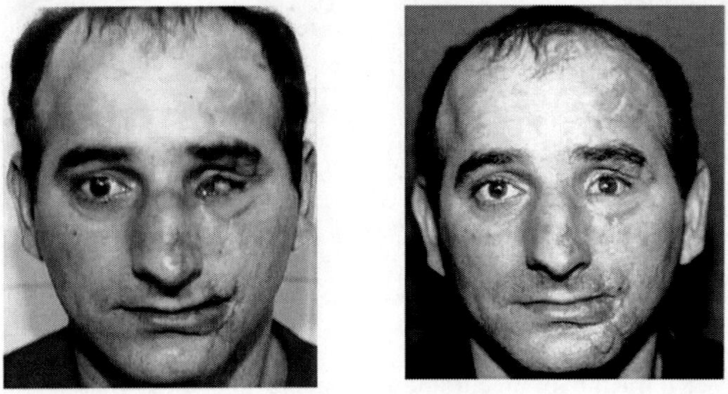

A B

Figure 18. A Injury of the orbit on the left with anophthalmos and defects of the orbital floor, infraorbital and lateral rims, and conjunctival sac. B. Condition of the patient after reconstruction of the conjunctival sac and orbital walls using rib cartilage. The contours of the face and orbit are normal, and conditions for good adaptation of the eye prosthesis are provided.

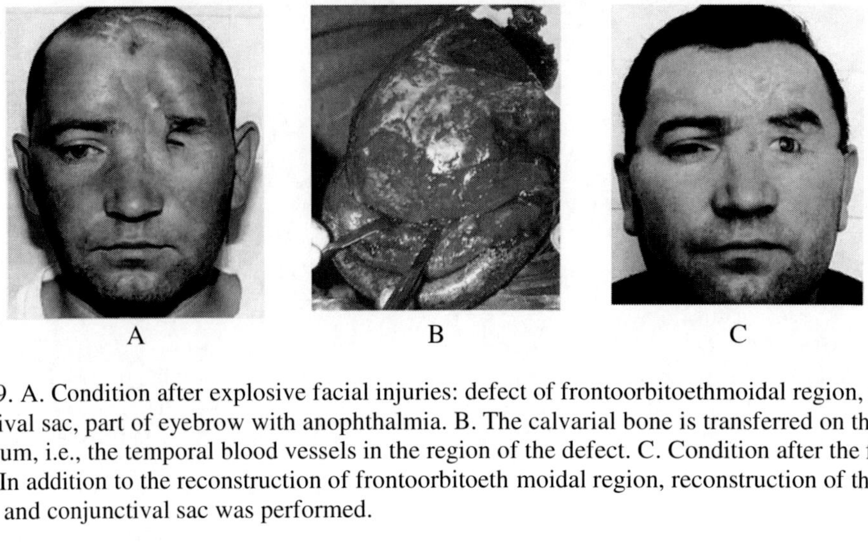

A B C

Figure 19. A. Condition after explosive facial injuries: defect of frontoorbitoethmoidal region, eyelids, conjunctival sac, part of eyebrow with anophthalmia. B. The calvarial bone is transferred on the pericranium, i.e., the temporal blood vessels in the region of the defect. C. Condition after the first surgery. In addition to the reconstruction of frontoorbitoeth moidal region, reconstruction of the eyelids, eyebrow and conjunctival sac was performed.

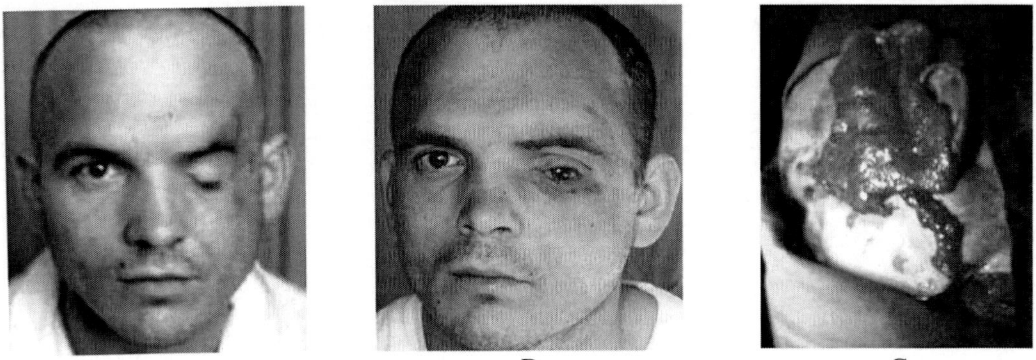

A B C

Figure 20. A. Neglected war injuries. A defect of the temporal and zygomatic regions as well as the orbital walls with anophthalmos. B. The orbital walls were reconstructed using rib cartilage, the facial contours were corrected using a deepithelialized forearm flap transferred with microsurgical techniques. Concomitantly, the lower eyelid and conjunctival sac were reconstructed. It is necessary to replace the prosthesis and put a new bigger prosthesis. C. Deepithelialized forearm flap simulates future position in the subcutaneous space.

2.5. Patients and Surgical Therapy Results

Of the 130 injured in the area of eye sockets, 86 persons had fresh injuries and 44 had neglected injuries (Table 1). In the cases of recent orbital fractures (Figures 3-9), after the reposition of the orbital contents, the reconstruction of orbital shape and volume, that is repair of the orbital bone defects, was performed using variety of material such as: the anterior wall of the maxillary sinus, outer cortex of the chin, iliac or calvarial bone, the rib cartilage graft and the silastic sheet. With all the above materials were obtained similar results. Silastik sheet is used only in 4 patients. In one patient due to rejection of silastik material, after removal of silastik sheet rib cartilage graft was used.

In cases of neglected fractures (Figures 10-20) it is necessary to perform refracture of the bone, reposition and fixation of the bone fragments and than reconstruction of the orbital shape and volume. This was achieved with the use of thick, formed rib cartilage graft in most cases. The neglected fractures of the midface were previously osteomized with the reposition and fixation of the bone fragments.

Detailed evaluation of the results in relation to the postoperative enophtalmos, diplopia and impaired sensibility of infraorbital region was performed in 72 patients (Table 2). From these results it can be seen that in the case of fresh orbital injuries significantly better results are achieved compared to the neglected injuries.

Table 1. Patients with orbital fractures

▪	Recent fractures	86
▪	Neglected fractures	44
▪	TOTAL	130

Table 2. Postoperative results regarding enophthalmos, diplopia and infraorbital nerve disturbance

	Enophthalmos			Diplopia			Infraorbital nerve disturbance		
		Postop.		Preop.	Postop.			Postop.	
	Preop	discrete	evident		straight gaze	lateral and/or upward gaze	Preop.	hypostesia	anesthesia
Group 1	20	3	2	14	-	2	18	4	3
Group 2	20	2	-	17	-	-	9	-	-
Group 3	25	7	3	18	3	6	20	8	4
Group 4	7	2	2	5	1	1	4	1	-
TOTAL	72	14	7	54	4	9	51	13	7

Conclusion

Traumatic fractures of the orbit are fairly frequent injuries both in wartime and in peacetime. Most often they are part of facial injuries but they can also be isolated. They are followed by numerous symptoms such as eye dislocation, enophthalmos, double vision, and often by various injuries of eye accessory organs. The conservative treatment of these injuries has been mostly abandoned. Surgical therapy – that is the reconstruction of the original orbital shape and volume as well as repositioning of orbital contents to their previous position—has to be performed as soon as possible. In cases of neglected fractures it is necessary to refracture the bone, reposition and fix the broken orbital fragments, and then, concomitantly, reconstruct the orbital shape and volume as well as reposition the orbital contents in their original position. In patients with neglected injuries, results of surgical treatment (i.e., correction of eye position, enophthalmos, and double vision) are considerably poorer than those achieved after the surgical treatment of fresh injuries.

References

[1] Bite U., Jackson I.T., Forbest G.S., Gehring D.G., Orbital volume measurements in enophthalmos using three-dimensional CT imaging. *Plast. Reconstr. Surg.* 75: 502-507, 1985.

[2] Converse J.M., Smith B., Enophthalmos and diplopia fracture of the orbital floor. *Br. J. Plast. Surg*. 9: 265-269, 1957.

[3] Converse J.M., Smith B., Obear M.F., Wood-Smith D.: Orbital blowout fractures: A ten-year study *Plast. Reconstr. Surg*. 39: 20-25, 1967.

[4] Converse J.M., Smith B., Wood-Smith D., Orbital and nasoorbital fractures. In: Converse J.M.: Reconstructive Plastic Surgery, Saunders Company, Philadelphia, 748-793, 1977.

[5] Crikelair G.F., Rein J.M., Potter G.D., Cosman B., A critical look at the blowout fracture. *Plast. Reconstr. Surg.* 49: 374-379, 1972.

[6] Dingman R.O., Converse J.M., The clinical management of facial injuries and fractures of the facial bones, In: Converse J.M.: Reconstructive Plastic Surgery, W.B. Saunders Company, Philadelphia, 599-747,1977.

[7] Dingman R.O., Natvig P., Surgery of facial fractures. W.B. Saunders Company, Philadelphia, 1964.

[8] Emery J.M., Noorden G.K., Schlernitzauer D.A., Management of orbital floor fractures. *Am.J. Ophthalmol.* 74: 299-306, 1972.

[9] Fujino T., Makino K. Entrapment mechanism and ocular injury in orbital blowout fracture. *Plast. Reconstr. Surg.* 65: 571-574, 1980.

[10] Horiono B., Recent correspondence on blow-out fracture. Intersectional meeting, Military Medical Academy, Belgrade, 1983.

[11] Hotte H.H., *Orbital fractures*. Van Gorcum, Assen, 1970.

[12] Jordan D.R., Onge P.S., Adrson R.L., Patrinely J.R., Nerad J. A.: Complications associated with alloplastic implants used in orbital floor fracture repair. *Ophthalmology* 99: 1600-1608, 1992.

[13] Kawamoto H.K., Late posttraumatic enophthalmos: A correctable deformity. *Plast. Reconstr. Surg.* 69: 423-427, 1982.

[14] Kohn R., Romano P., E., Pulkin J.E., Lacrimal obstruction after migration of orbital floor implant *Am. J. Ophthalmol.* 82: 934-936, 1976.

[15] Koorneef L., Current concepts on the management of orbital blowout fractures. *Ann. Plast. Surg.* 9: 185-200, 1982.

[16] Koorneef L., Sectional anatomy of the orbit. Aeolus Press, Amsterdam, 1981.

[17] Lireman I.R., Loss vision associated with surgical treatment of zygomatic orbital floor fracture. *Plast. Reconstr. Surg.* 68: 94-97, 1981.

[18] Longarce J.J., Kahl J.B., Wood R.W., Reconstruction of extensive defects in and about the orbit. *Am. J. Ophthalmol.* 61: 763-768, 1996.

[19] Manson P.N., Clifford M.A., Iliff N.T., Morgan R., Mechanisms of global support and posttraumatic enophthalmos: I. The anatomy of the ligamentsling and its relation to intramuscular cone orbital fat. *Plast. Reconstr. Surg.* 77: 193-202, 1986.

[20] Manson P.N, Grivas A., Rosenbaum A., Vannier M., Zinreich J., Iliff N., Studies on Enophthalmos: II. The measurement of orbital injuries. *Plast. Reconstr. Surg.* 77; 203-214, 1986.

[21] Manson P.N., Iliff M.T., Post-traumatic orbitl repositioning. In: Toth B.A., Keating R.E., Stewart W.B., ed. An atlas of orbitocranial surgery. Martin Dunitz, London, 1999, 182-202.

[22] Manson P.N., Raus E.J., Iliff N.T., Deep orbital reconstruction for correction of posttraumatic enophthalmos. *Clin. Plast. Surg.*14: 113-121, 1987.

[23] Mauriello J.A., Fiore P.M., Kotch M., Dacryocystitis: late complication of orbital floor fracture repair with implant. *Ophthalmology* 94: 248-250, 1987.

[24] Mauriello J.A., Hargrave S., Mostafavi R., Kapila R., Infection after insertion of alloplastics orbital floor impants. *Am. J. Ophthalmol.* 117: 246-252, 1994.

[25] Mustarde J.C., Repair and reconstruction in the orbital region: A practical guide. Churchill Livingstone, Edinburgh, 1980.

[26] Mustarde J.C., The role of the Lockwood's suspensoru ligament in preventing downward displacement of the eye. *Br. J. Plast. Surg*. 21:73-81, 1968.

[27] Nicholson D.H., Guzak S.V., Visual loss complicating repair orbital floor fractures. *Arch. Ophtahalmol.* 86: 369-375, 1971.

[28] Ortiz-Monasterio F., Rodrigez A., Benavides A., A simple method for the correction of enophthalmos. *Clin. Plast. Surg*. 14: 169-175, 1987.

[29] Putterman A.M., Stevens T., Urist M.J., Nonsurgical management of blowour fractures of the orbital floor. *Am. J. Ophthalmol*. 77: 232-239, 1974.

[30] Reny A., Striker M., Fractures de l'orbite. Indications ophthalmologiques dans les techniques operatories. Masson & Cie, Paris, 1969.

[31] Rončević R., Reconstruction of internal orbital fractures. *Plast. Reconstr. Surg*. 89:1176-1177,1992.

[32] Roncevic R., Discussion on ''Lactosorb panel and screw for repair of large orbital floor defects''. *J. Cranio-Maxillofac. Surg*. 26: 191-192, 1998.

[33] Rončević R., Refracture of untreated fractures of the zygomatic bone. *J. Max-Fac. Surg*. 11: 252-256, 1983.

[34] Rončević R., Malinger B.: The validity of certain metods of reposition of zygomatic bone. Vojnosanitetski pregled 36:23-25,1979.

[35] Rončević R., Malinger B., Experience with various procedures in the treatment of orbital floor fractures. *J. Max-Fac. Surg*.9: 81-84, 1981.

[36] Rončević R., Osvald M., Popovič M., The possibility of radiological diagnostics in maxillofacial region. *Chirurgia maxillofac.-plastica* 11:47-54,1980.

[37] Rončević R., Rončević D., Extensive, traumatic fractures of the orbit in war and peace time. *J. Craniofac. Surg*. 10: 284-300, 1999.

[38] Rončević R., Stajčić Z., Surgical treatment of posttraumatic enophthalmos: A study of 72 patients. *Ann. Plast. Surg*. 32: 288-294, 1994.

[39] Rončević R., Stajčić Z., Surgical treatment of posttraumatic enophthalmos. In: Home Study Course, Plastic and Reconstructive Problems, American Academy of Head and Neck Surgery Foundantion, Inc., p.279-285, 1996.

[40] Rumelt M.B., Ernest J.T., Isolated blowout fracture of the medial orbital wall with medial rectus entrapment. *Am. J. Ophthalmol*. 73: 451-455, 1972.

[41] Sacks A.C., Friedland J.A., Orbital fractures. Should they be explored early. *Plast. Reconstr. Surg*. 64: 190-193, 1979.

[42] Smith B., Regan W.F. Jr., Blowout fracture of the orbit: Mechanism and correction of internal orbital fractures. *Am. J. Ophthalmol*. 44: 733-739, 1957.

[43] Tenzel R.R., Miller G.R., Orbital blowout fracture repair, conjunctival approach. *Am. J. Ophthalmol*. 71: 1141-1142, 1971.

[44] Tessier P., The conjunctival approach in orbital fractures. *Plast. Reconst. Surg*. 52: 656-659, 1973.

[45] Yano H., Nakano M., Anraku K. et al.: A consecutuve review of orbital blowout fractures and recommendations for comprehensive management *Plast. Reconst. Surg*. 124:602-611, 2009.

Chapter 3

Surgery of the Orbital Tumors

3.1. Introduction

There is a large number of tumors in the eye, the eye adnexa, the orbit and the surrounding regions, requiring a minor or a major surgical procedure. It is not the aim of this book to present all the data and information about the origin, pathogenesis, type, classification, clinical picture, diagnostics and treatment of all the tumors. Having in mind that many books and articles (1-34), were written about this topic, this book shall elaborate only the most essential facts, but with detailed descriptions of surgical procedures in the orbital region.

3.2. Basic Classification of Orbital Tumors

Orbital tumors can be primary or secondary; both can be benign or malign. The most frequent primary benign orbital tumors are hemangiomas, dermoid cysts, eosinophilic granuloma, meningioma, various fibromas, osteomas, lipomas, tumors of neural origin and teratomas. The most frequent primary malignant orbital tumors are malignant lymphoma [1, 2, 5, 16, 25] and various sarcomas. The lacrimal gland and the lacrimal sac are both located in the orbit. The most widespread benign tumors of the lacrimal gland are adenomas, and the most frequent malignant tumors are adenocarcinomas and malignant mixtus tumors. Papillomas are the most frequent benign tumors of the lacrimal sac, whereas squamocellular carcinomas are the most widespread malignant tumors.

Secondary orbital tumors can reach the orbit from the surrounding regions *per continuitatem* or from the distant regions as metastasis. Most of the secondary orbital tumors are actually the advanced-stage tumors from the surrounding regions [3, 7, 17]. Most often those are basocellular and squamocellular carcinomas of the eyelids, sinuses, nose, nasopharynx, conjunctiva, infratemporal, frontal and temporal region [27]. The benign tumors of the surrounding regions, most often osteomas and chondromas, rarely reach the orbit. Metastatic secondary orbital tumors [10, 12] are rare and most often those are breast and lung cancers. The secondary orbital tumors also include various intraocular tumors, which penetrate the solid fibrous corneoscleral membrane and enter the orbit, or even metastase outside the orbit. These are most often tumors of uvea and retina. The malignant melanoma of the uvea is the most widespread intraocular tumor. Retinoblastoma, which is also very malignant, is quite scarce.

Various inflammatory lesions similar to tumors can also appear in the orbit [6, 20, 25, 30, 34] such as the inflammatory pseudotumor, Wegener's granulomatosis, sarcoidosis, nodular fasciitis, multifocal sclerosing inflammatory lesion, lipogranuloma, mucocele of the paranasal sinuses etc. All the above-mentioned conditions can produce a clinical picture of the orbital tumor.

The orbit and the orbital content can be affected and even destroyed by tumor-like diseases, such as neurofibromatosis and fibrous dysplasia of the facial bones and the skull [26]. These diseases can be found in the orbit either as the primary or the secondary lesions.

3.3. Clinical Picture of the Orbital Tumor

The clinical picture of the orbital tumors is quite diverse and depends on the type, size and the location of the tumor. The primary tumors cause an increase in the volume of the orbital content, which results in the eyeball protrusion that is most often referred to as the exophthalmos or proptosis (Figures 10, 11, 19, 21). Exophthalmos is more pronounced when the tumor is located in the retrobulbar part of the orbit. Dislocation of the eyeball is almost a regular occurrence in primary orbital tumors (Figures 10, 11, 21). The eyeball is moved to the opposite of the tumor infiltrating side. The tumors in the upper part of the orbit move the eye downwards, whereas tumors in the medial part of the orbit move the eyeball sideways. The primary orbital tumors are rarely localized at the orbital floor. The upward dislocation of the eye indicates a process that penetrated the orbit from the maxillary sinus. The eye dislocation is greater if the tumor is located in the anterior part of the orbit. The gazes are usually limited towards the direction of the tumor. Restriction of the eyeball movements is quite conspicuous when the malignant orbital tumors infiltrate the bulbomotor muscles (Figure 21). In larger orbital tumors most often both the exophthalmos and the eyeball dislocation can be observed (Figures 10, 11, 21). The exophthalmos and dislocation of the bulbus are frequently accompanied by strabismus and diplopia (Figures 10, 11, 19). The primary orbital tumors can be accompanied by various degrees of vision loss depending on the type, localization and the size of the tumor.

The secondary metastatic orbital tumors, as well as the intraocular tumors penetrating the orbit, can produce a similar clinical picture as the primary orbital tumors. Naturally, the loss of vision most often occurs in cases of intraocular tumors. The secondary orbital tumors which penetrate the orbit from the surrounding regions *per continuitatem,* may also be accompanied, depending on the localization, type and size, by all manifestations of the primary orbital tumors, such as swelling, inflammation, deformities, ulcerations and necrosis of the surrounding regions, the eyelids and the conjunctiva (Figures 15, 16, 18, 21, 22).

3.4. Orbital Tumor Diagnosis

Anamnesis provides the information about the start and the course of the illness and the chief symptoms. Gradual occurrence of the unilateral exophthalmos, without any other signs, is the characteristic of the benign orbital tumors. Sudden occurrence of exophthalmos, accompanied by swelling of the surrounding tissue can occur mainly in the orbital inflammatory pseudotumors. The suffusion of the eyelids, followed by exophthalmos, can be the first sign of the malignant tumor. Pain is not characteristic for the primary orbital tumors and it rarely occurs (20). It is more frequent in cases of inflammatory pseudotumors. The secondary tumors, which penetrate the orbit from the surrounding regions *per continuitatem* are usually accompanied with a more severe pain. Inspection is sufficient to note the occurrence of exophthalmos, the eyeball dislocation, primary position and eye motility, eye pulsation, as well as the pathological changes in cornea, conjunctiva, the eyelids and the surrounding structures. Palpation is used to feel the lesions in the anterior and central part of the orbit, as well as infiltration of the malignant tumors in the anterior part of the orbit and the surrounding regions. Sensitivity to touch and the degree of resistance to palpation pressure cannot provide much assistance in reaching the diagnosis [20]. A routine ophthalmological examination can provide information about the visual acuity, visual field, eye fundus and the intraocular pressure. The degree of exophthalmos can be determined by Hertel exophthalmometry. Occurrence of diplopia is more accurately determined by the Hess-Lancaster test. Roentgenography (native and contrast) provides important information about the position, size and the type of tumor [28].

Modern powerful diagnostic devices, such as echography (ultrasonography), computed tomography (CT), tridimensional computed tomography (3D-CT) and magnetic resonance imaging (MRI), provide an extraordinary orbital tumor diagnostics, i.e., give information about their size, position, morphological characteristics, topographic relation to important structures of the eye and the orbit, and also about the nature of the pathological process. In some cases, when the above-mentioned methods of diagnostics fail to provide convincing diagnosis, orbital scintigraphy can be tried. The final preoperative diagnosis about the nature of the pathological process can be obtained with biopsy, including aspiration biopsy.

3.5. Orbital Tumor Therapy

Only after a proper diagnosis is reached is it possible to determine the therapy. The orbital tumor therapy can be surgical, radiological and chemotherapeutical. These three methods of therapy are often combined.

3.5.1. Irradiation Therapy

The orbital irradiation therapy represents unique problem as two basic principles of the therapy must be satisfied in the small space of the orbit: a tumoricidal dosage of radiation has to be applied, while the surrounding healthy tissues, that are very radiosensitive, have to be spared from damage and functional impairment.

Irradiation therapy is the therapy of choice in cases of lymphoid orbital tumors – benign, of uncertain nature, or malignant. In case of malignant lymphoma this therapy is often combined with polychemotherapy. Diagnostic biopsy is the only surgical intervention applied to any lymphoid lesion of the orbit and the conjunctiva [20].

The irradiation therapy is also indicated in plasmocytoma, myeloma, eosinophilic granuloma, and even in some intraocular tumors such as retinoblastoma. The irradiation therapy is most often applied after the surgical therapy in primary or secondary malignant orbital tumors, particularly following exenteration of the orbit.

3.5.2. Polychemotherapy

In certain instances surgical or irradiation therapy can be combined with polychemotherapy. Polychemotherapy is most often applied in orbital systemic diseases (tumors) of hematopoietic or lymphoid origin. Inflammatory pseudotumors are treated with corticosteroids and immunosuppressants, and occasionally with surgical and irradiation therapy.

3.5.3. Surgical Therapy

Surgical therapy of the orbital tumors is the most effective therapy. Depending on the type, localization and the size, the tumor can be removed by excision, i.e., by tumor extirpation or by exenteration of the orbit. Intraocular tumors, depending on their type, localization and size can be removed by excision, evisceration or enucleation. This book shall not discuss these purely ophthalmological surgical procedures.

Bony margins and the orbital walls significantly hinder the access to the orbital tumors. With development of craniofacial surgery, the approach to pathological processes of the orbit has been improved, so that nowadays significant surgical results are being achieved. Depending on the type, localization and the size of the tumor, it can be removed by orbitotomy without removing the bone [11, 18], orbitotomy with temporary marginectomy, i.e., temporary removal of the orbital margins [18, 29, 32, 33], or ostectomy – temporary or permanent removal of certain margins and walls of the orbit [9, 15, 21, 22, 24, 31].

Surgical interventions in the orbit, with different scope and complexity, range from ordinary incisions and excisions with direct closures, up to complex approaches with exploration of the orbit, intracranial space and paranasal sinuses, with extensive resections of soft and bone tissues. These extensive resections of the tissue cause major defects, which require complicated reconstructive procedures of the bone and soft tissues in order to obtain acceptable functional and aesthetic results.

3.5.3.1. Anterior Orbitotomy

Anterior orbitotomy implies the approach to the orbit, i.e., perirobital space through skin or the conjunctive (Figures 1-6). Basically, the anterior orbitotomy without removal of the bone margins or walls of the orbit provides access to all the lesions in the anterior half of the orbit [11, 18, 22]. Indications for anterior orbitotomy are: drainage, biopsy, tumor removal, decompression of the orbit, reconstruction of the orbital walls and rehabilitation of the orbital fracture. Depending on the lesion position, the anterior orbitotomy can be performed by medial, superior, inferior and lateral approach.

Medial Approach

Depending on the size, position and type of lesion, the medial space of the orbit can be approached by the coronal (Lynch) approach (Figure 1), conjunctival extraconal or conjunctival intraconal approach (Figure 2). Coronal (Lynch) approach represents an incision from the medial part of the eyebrow, which incision descends above the base of the nasal pyramid towards the base of nasal ala (Figure 1). The incision can be extended laterally below the eyebrow, or through the eyebrow, to the end of the eyebrow. After the incision of the skin and the subcutaneous tissue, the periosteum is cut in front of the anterior lacrimal crest. This is followed by a wide lifting of the periosteum with the lifting of the lacrimal sac from its fossa. The medial canthal ligament is lifted or separated from its annex on the anterior lacrimal crest. Such an approach allows exploration of the medial part of the orbit, the medial orbital wall, the medial part of the orbital roof and floor, the lacrimal sac and the lacrimal duct. This approach also enables performing of all the surgical procedures in the lacrimal sac and duct, including the dacryocystorhinostomy. The sphenoid sinus can be approached through the posterior part of the ethmoid sinus. By this approach through the sphenoid sinus it is possible to perform decompression of the optic nerve.

The most frequent indications for this type of approach are mucocele and other sinus lesions penetrating the orbit, as well as the pathology of the lacrimal sac and the lacrimal duct. In order to remove the ethmoid part of the medial orbital wall, for the purpose of orbital decompression in the events of dysthyroid ophthalmopathy, a short incision, descending from the medial part of the eyebrow to the level of the medial corner of the eye, shall be sufficient. In the course of this procedure neither the lacrimal sac nor the medial ligament should be lifted.

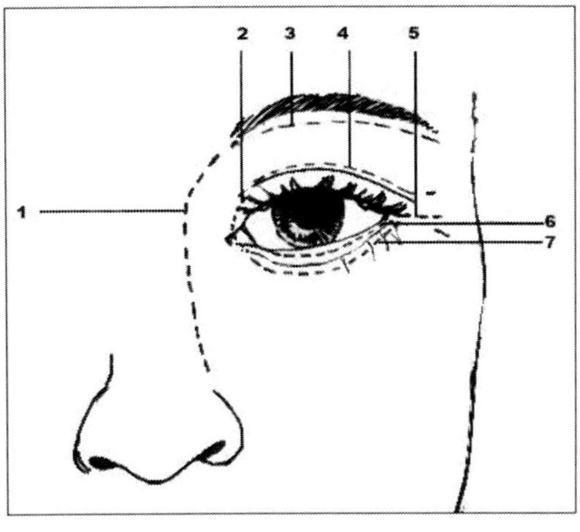

Figure 1. Incisions – approaches to anterior orbitotomy: 1. – Lynch approach, 2. – Medial conjunctival approach, 3. – Approach through the eyebrow, 4. – Approach through the upper eyelid, 5. – Approach through the lateral cantus, 6. – Inferior conjunctival approach, 7. – Subciliary approach.

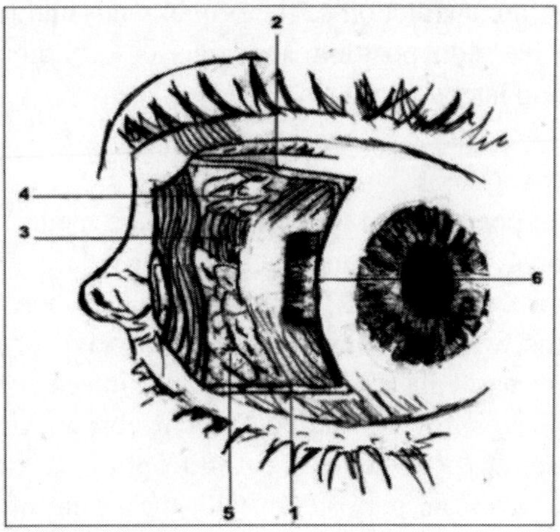

Figure 2. Medial conjunctival intraconal approach: 1,2 - Conjuctival incisions, 3 – Optic nerve, 4,5 – Intraconal fat tissue, 6 – Part of medial rectus muscle.

For the conjunctival extraconal approach the incision is applied through the medial conjunctiva. The incision can be expanded into the superior and inferior conjunctival fornix. The entrance to the orbit is behind the lacrimal sac. This approach allows exploration of the medial wall and the medial part of the orbital floor, as well as of trochlea and the tendon of the superior oblique muscle. For the conjunctival intraconal approach (Figure 2) the vertical incision is performed close to the cornea margin, and then two horizontal parallel incisions are made medially to the end. After lifting the conjunctival flap, the medial rectus muscle is cut close to its insertion to the bulbus. After this, it is possible to approach the anterior part of the retrobulbar intraconal space formed by the extraocular rectus muscles, which is filled with the fat tissue.

Superior Approach

For the superior approach, the incision can be applied on the upper eyelid groove (Figure 1), along the eyebrow (supraciliary incision) or directly beneath the eyebrow (Figures 1, 3), as well as the the coronal incision in the hairy part of the temporal and the frontal region (Figure 8). If the orbit is approached by incision at the palpebral groove, in order to penetrate the retrobulbar intraconal space, the aponeurosis of the upper eyelid levator muscle must be cut. If this incision is used for entering below the orbital roof, dissection can be made leaving the orbital septum intact. In order to facilitate the inspection of the superior part of the orbit and to allow surgical procedure, it is sometimes necessary to take the supraorbital neurovascular bundle, by careful dissection, out of its groove or canal and move it medially. The incision in the supraciliary region, along the eyebrow or directly beneath the eyebrow (Figure 1) allows a wider and direct approach to the superior part of the orbit. Naturally, the supraorbital and the supratrochlear neurovascular bundle must be preserved with this incision also. For a better survey of the superior part of the orbit, temporary marginectomy of the superior orbital margin can be performed (Figure 4), with preserving the above mentioned neurovascular bundles. Upon the completion of the surgical procedure in the orbit, the bony fragment of the orbital margin shall be returned to its original position and fixed by a stainless steel wire 0.4 mm thick, or by mini i.e., micro plates. The coronal incision in the hairy part of the temporal and the frontal region (Figure 8) requires a larger tissue dissection, and in bald men it leaves a visible scar.

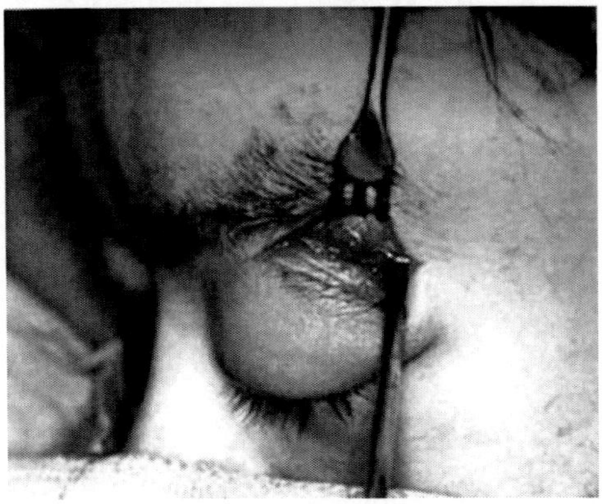

Figure 3. Transcutane superior approach for the anterior orbitotomy. The tumor protrudes under the superior orbital margin.

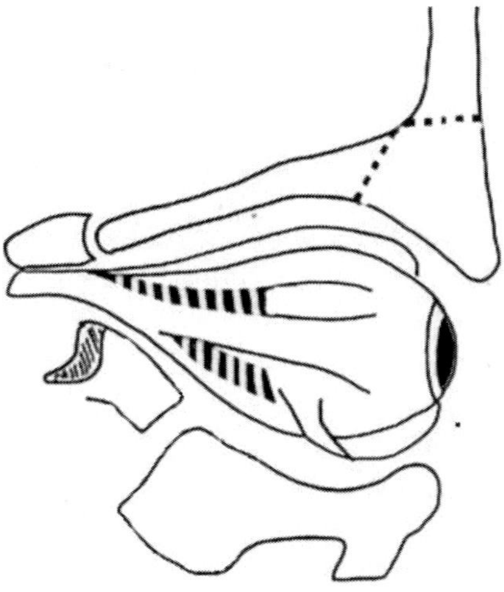

Figure 4. Diagram of superior marginotomy.

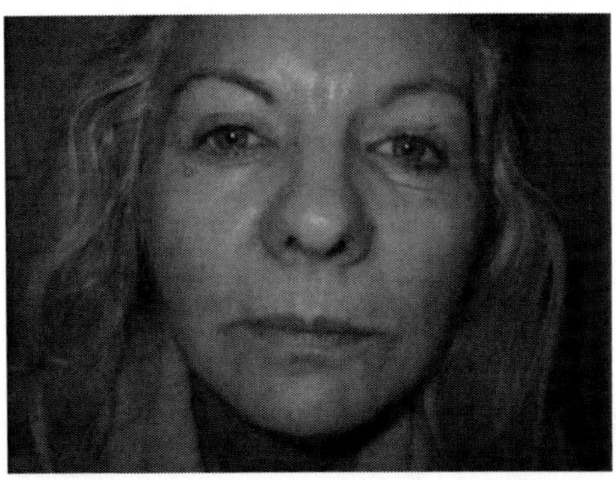

Figure 5. Approaches for the lower anterior orbitotomy on the lower eyelid: a – subciliary, b – lower subciliary, c – palpebral-orbital.

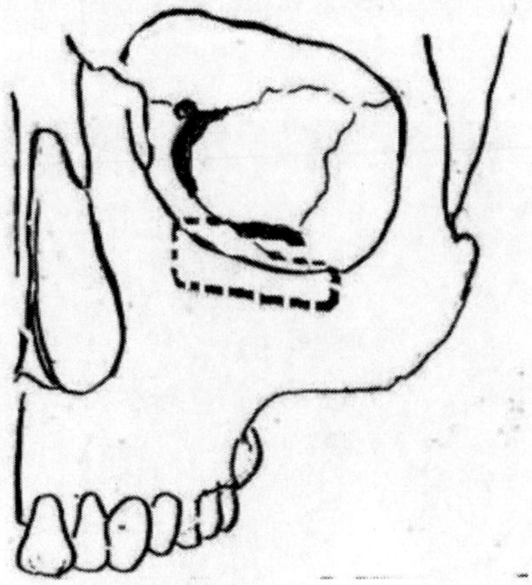

Figure 6. Diagram of lower inferior marginotomy.

Inferior Approach

Inferior approach can be made through an incision at the conjunctive or at the lower eyelid (Figure 1). A wider, better approach is provided by a subciliary incision at the lower eyelid (Figure 5) that leaves almost an invisible scar. After the incision, the skin is separated from the muscle up to the level of the infraorbital margin, and then this margin is reached by the incision through the muscle. After the incision of the periosteum on the orbital margin, the periosteum is lifted from the floor and the lateral orbital wall. When performing this dissection the infraorbital neurovascular bundle should be preserved.

This approach allows exploration of the inferior orbital margin, the orbital floor, the lateral orbital margin, the lateral orbital wall, the part of the medial orbital wall and the extraconal part of the lower lateral part of the orbit. For the purpose of visualization in the area of the orbital apex and the inferior orbital fissure, temporary marginectomy of the inferior orbital margin can be performed (Figure 6). After the operation, this bony fragment shall be returned to its original position and fixed by a stainless steel wire 0.4 mm thick, or by mini i.e., micro plates.

Lateral Approach

The lateral approach is performed by an incision through the lateral part of the superior and the inferior conjunctival fornix or by the skin incision in the region of the lateral part of the eyebrow (Figure 7). Both mentioned methods enable surgical procedures in the anterior part of the lateral part of the orbit. Disinsertion of the lateral ligament provides a better survey and a wider approach to the pathological processes. After the operation, the reinsertion of the lateral ligament must be performed by connecting it to the periosteum or to the orbital margin by previously drilling a hole into the bone.

3.5.3.2. Lateral Orbitotomy

The removal of the lateral orbital wall for the purpose of exploring the orbit and removing the pathological lesion was first described by Kronlein in 1888. This approach has been quite used nowadays. For approaching the lateral wall of the orbit, most often applies a skin incision at the level of the lateral orbital margin, which descends to the level of the lateral corner of the eye, and then is extended laterally and downwards by 1 cm along the natural groove (Figure 7). It is also possible to use Burke's incision (4), i.e., a horizontal incision from the lateral corner of the eye, about 2 cm long (Figure 7).

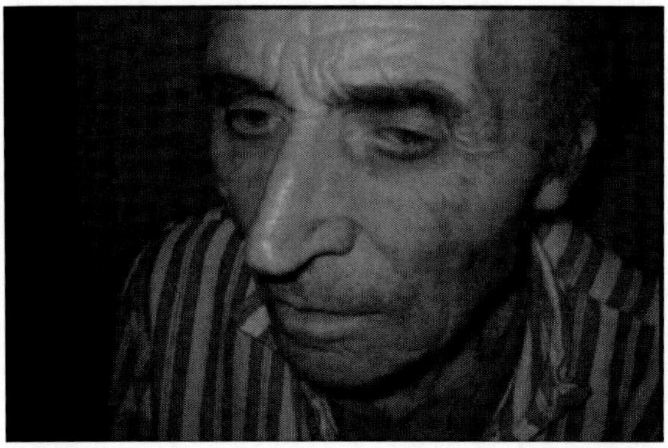

Figure 7. Approach for lateral orbitotomy: a – incision at the level of the lateral orbital margin, b – horizontal incision.

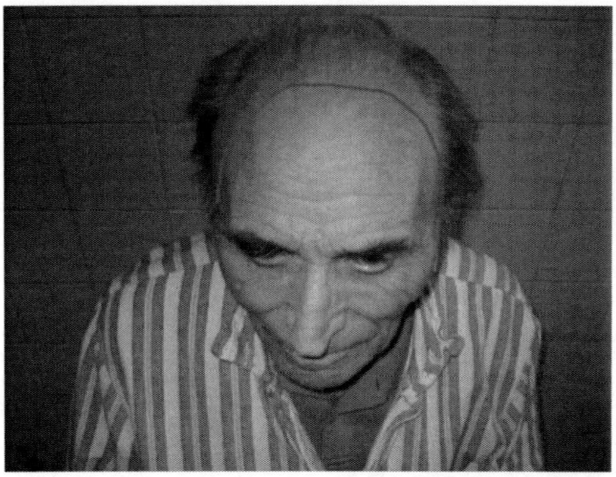

Figure 8. Coronal incision.

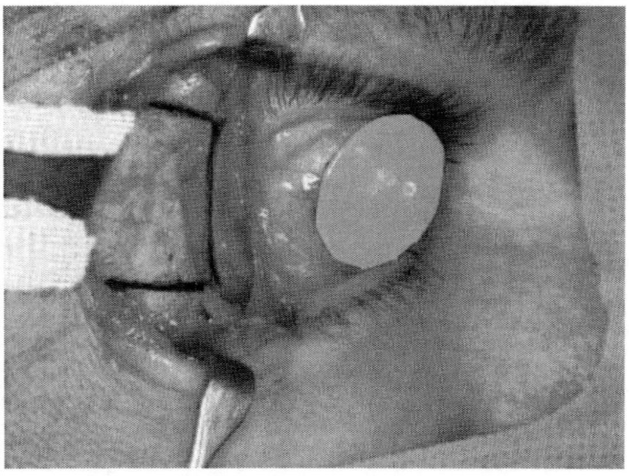

Figure 9. Explored lateral orbital wall and marked places of osteotomy.

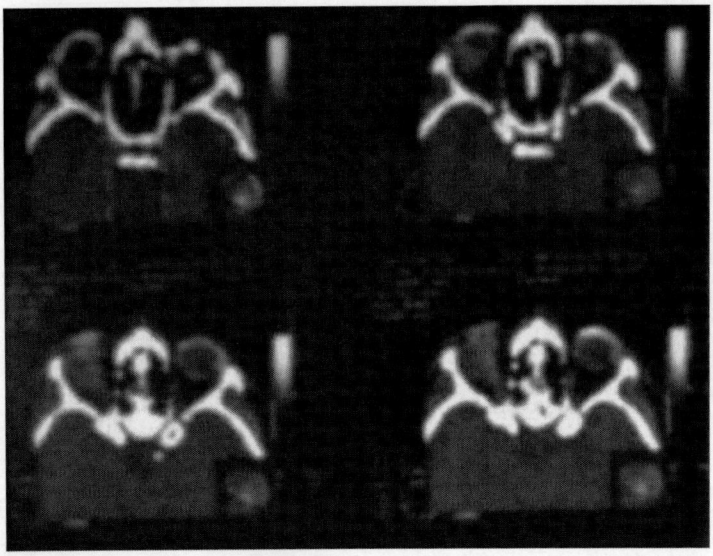

A

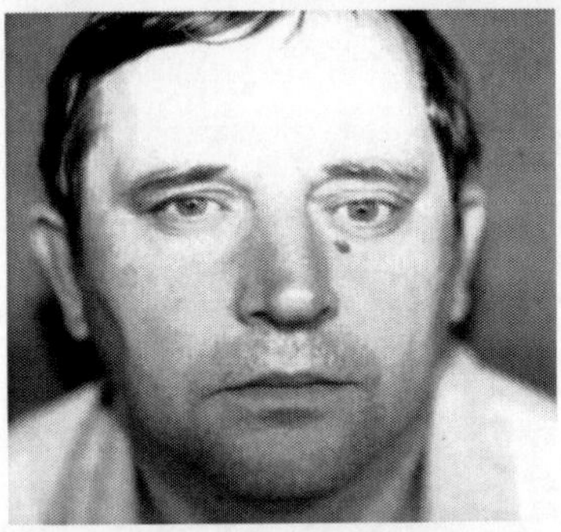

B

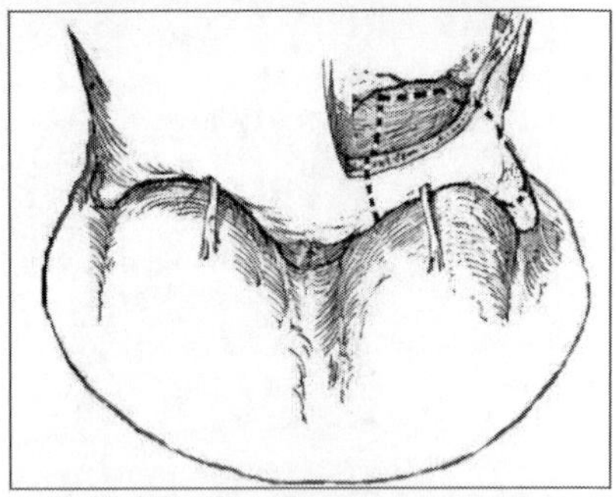

C

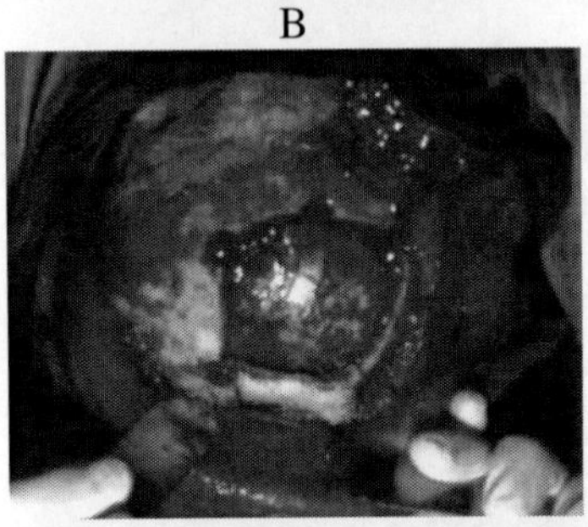

D

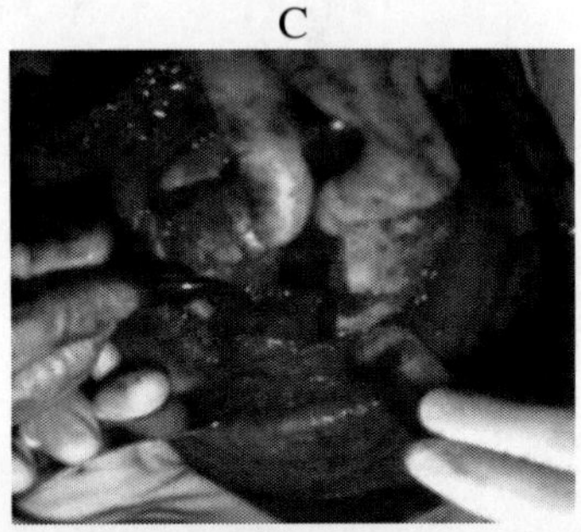

E

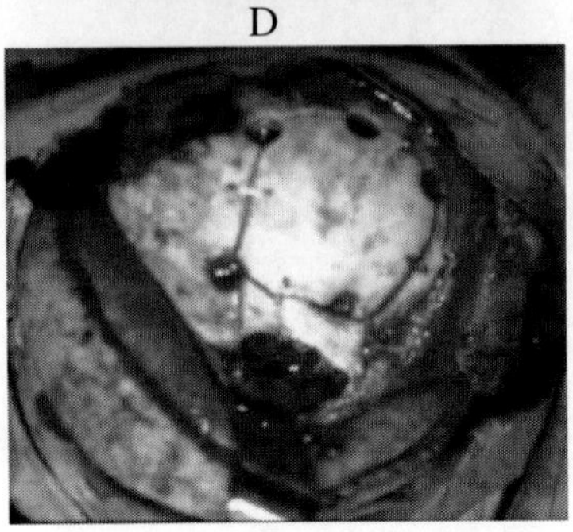

F

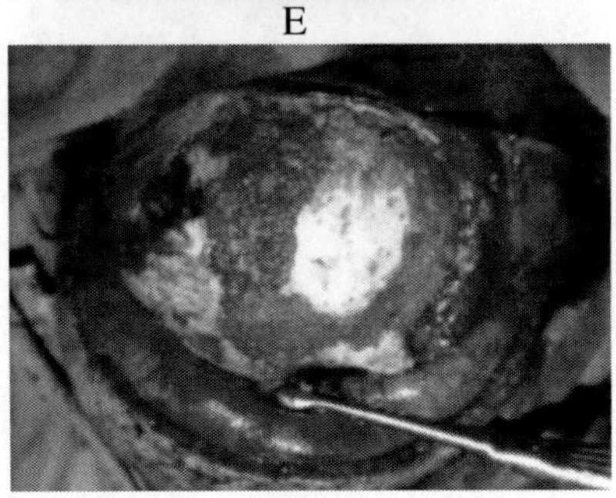

G

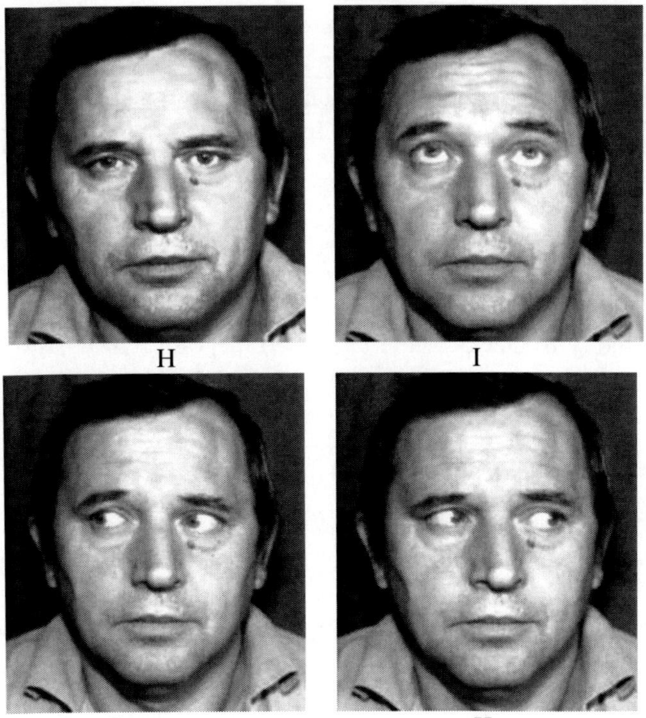

H I

J K

Figure 10. A, B. The patient with a tumor in the left superior and lateral retrobulbar part of the orbit, with the exophthalmos, bulbus dislocation and diplopias. C. A drawing of the supraorbital orbitotomy. D. After coronal incision and dissection of the soft tissues from the bones, a temporary ostectomy of the part of the frontal bone has been performed by a neurosurgical technique, i.e., a "window" has been made. After lifting the base of the brain from the orbital roof, a temporary ostectomy of the superior orbital margin, the orbital roof, as well as of the part of the lateral margin and the wall has been performed in a block. E. Removal of the tumor. F-After tumor removal and hemostasis, the bone fragments of the orbit and of the frontal bone are returned to their original position and fixed by a wire ligature. G. Places where osteotomy was performed are filled with bone scrapings. H. The same patient three months after the surgery. The position of the bulbus is symmetrical and there is no deformity in the region of the forehead and the orbit. I. Looking up. J. Looking right. K. Looking left. Eye movements are normal in all directions and there is no double vision.

The widest approach for the removal of the lateral orbital wall is provided by the coronal incision in the hairy part of the temporal and the frontal region (Figures 8, 10c, 11c, 19c). This incision avoids visible postoperative scar. It is performed by cutting the skin and the subcutaneous tissue, and then cutting the periosteum along the orbital margin. The incision at the periosteum starts above the frontozygomatic suture and spreads to the anterior part of the zygomatic arch. The periosteum and the temporal muscle separate from the bone and moved laterally, and then the periosteum, at the internal side of the lateral orbital wall, also separates from the bone. Afterwards, a small electric saw or a suitable borer is used for making osteotomy cuts on the orbital wall. The upper cut is 5-10 mm above the frontozygomatic suture; if necessary, it can be even further. The lower cut is performed directly above the zygomatic arch. This osteotomy procedure cuts both the orbital margin and the bone of the lateral wall up to a certain depth – depending on the requirement. These two vertical parallel cuts are connected to a third horizontal cut at the orbital wall (Figure 9). After such an osteotomy, the bony fragment of the orbital wall is temporarily removed. During the performance of the osteotomy the orbital content should be protected by a suitable retractor, i.e., a spatula. In order to explore the orbital content, periorbit should be cut in several places. The most appropriate is a horizontal incision from front to back, at the level of the lacrimal gland, and above the external rectus muscle. This is followed by a careful dissection of the tissue for identifying all the structures, performing biopsy or removing a pathological lesion. This approach allows a successful removal of the pathological extraconal and intraconal lesions in the lateral part of the orbit. The lesions located medially from the optic nerve as well as the lesions in the orbital apex cannot be removed by this approach. After the operation and hemostasis, the bony fragment of the lateral orbital wall returns into its original position and it is fixed by a non-resorptive suture, a stainless steel wire, or by micro plates. If coronal incision has been applied, the temporal muscle should be returned to its original position and fixed in order to avoid an impression in the anterior part of the temporal region.

3.5.3.3. Transcranial Supraorbital Orbitotomy and Transfacial Approach

For this approach it is necessary to apply a coronal incision in the hairy part of the ipsilateral temporal region, spreading through the hairy part of the frontal region all the way to the vicinity of the opposite temporal region (Figures 8, 10c, 11c, 19c). This approach, which is often used in craniofacial surgery, is indicated for the removal of pathological lesions in the superior part of the orbit, particularly in its apical part, and for the removal of lesions of the orbital roof and the anterior cranial fossa [9, 15, 31, 33]. After performing a coronal incision, all soft tissues of the frontal and the temporal region are lifted up to the superior and lateral orbital margin. In the temporal region the temporal muscle with the periosteum is separated from the external side of the lateral orbital wall. Then mentioned orbital margins are stripped of periosteum, as well as superior and lateral orbital walls. During deperiostation of orbital margins and walls the supraorbital and supratrochlear neurovascular bundles must be preserved. This is followed by a frontal bone osteotomy in the supraorbital region (Figure 11c) performed by a neurosurgical trepan and craniotom. Osteotomized part of the bone is temporarily removed (Figures 10c, 11d). Through this "window" on the frontal bone, the base of the brain with dura is lifted from the orbital roof. Then, by using a small electric saw or a suitable borer, the osteotomy of the supraorbital region with the orbital roof and the superior part of the lateral orbital wall is performed. This bone fragment is also temporarily removed (Figures 10 d, e, 11e). After this procedure and after the incision of the periorbit, a complete survey of the superior part of the orbit, up to the apex, is enabled.

By careful dissection of the tissue, with the direct view of the entire surgical field, it is possible to identify all orbital structures (Figure 11g), to remove a tumor and ensure protection of all the orbital structures against injuries, as much as possible. After removal of the pathological lesion and after careful hemostasis, the orbital bony fragment is returned to its original position and fixed by a stainless steel wire or by mini i.e., micro plates (Figures 10f, 11h). The fragment of the frontal bone is also returned to its original position and fixed to the adjacent bone in the same manner (Figures 10f, 11h). The soft tissues are also returned to their original positions and stitched in the usual manner. Beneath the soft tissues and above the bone, a suction drainage should be placed that will remain there for about two days.

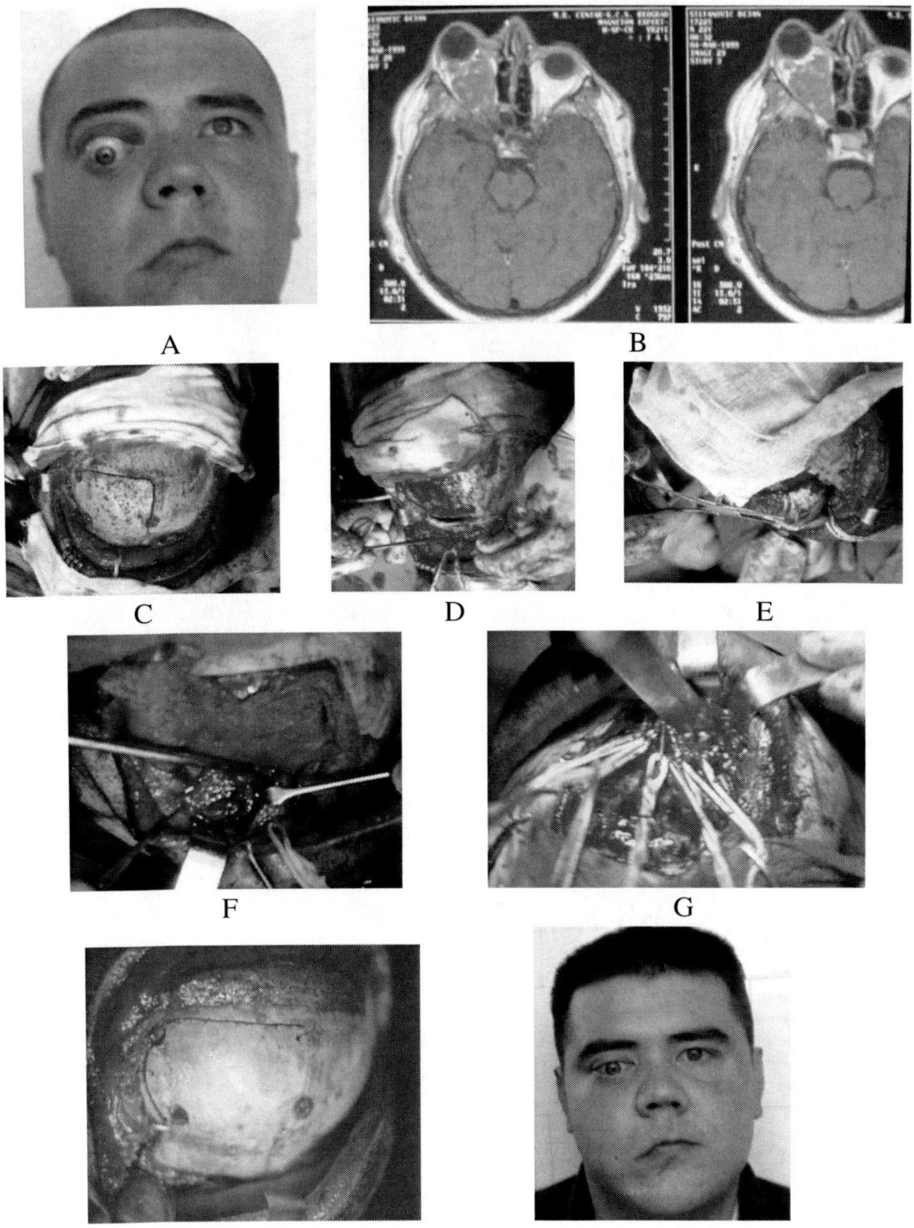

Figure 11. A. The patient with lymphhemangioma of the face and the right orbit, with excessive protrusion and dislocation of the right eye. B. An MRI image: the tumor fills in the entire orbit and the paraorbital space. C. Frontal bone osteotomy after a coronal incision. D. "Window" in the frontal bone through which the base of the brain is lifted from the orbital roof. The supraorbital neurovascular bundle has been lifted on a thin rubber band. E. After a supraorbital osteotomy, the superior orbital margin, the orbital roof and the superior part of the lateral orbital wall are temporarily removed in a block. F. By direct inspection of the entire surgical field, the entire superior part of the orbit and the tumor can be observed. G. The tumor has been removed and at the same time all orbital structures have been indicated. Bulbomotor muscles have been lifted on a thin rubber band. H. Bone fragments of the orbit and the frontal bone have been returned to their original position and fixed by a wire ligature. I. The same patient three months after the surgery: there are no visible deformities or scars on the forehead and in the orbital area.

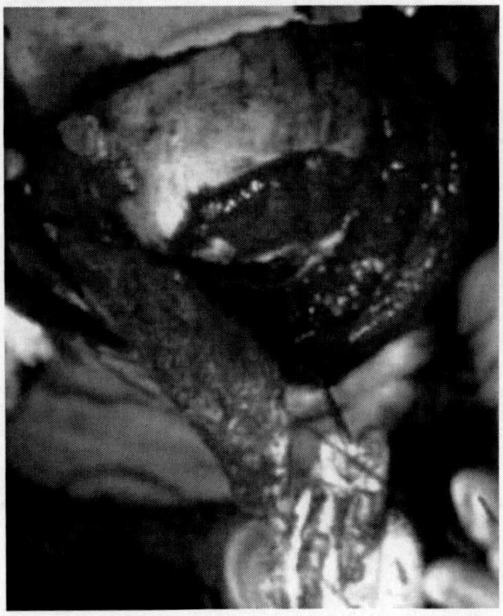

Figure 12. Pericranial, galeoperiosteal flap prepared for covering dura and the base of the brain.

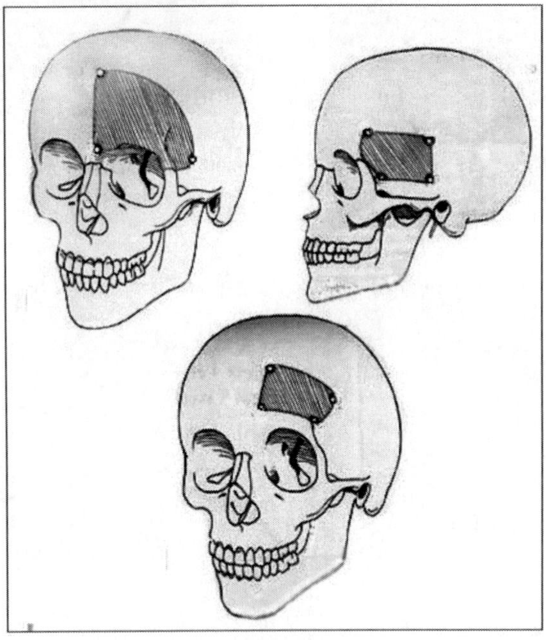

Figure 13. Neurosurgical, transcranial approaches to the orbit.

If the tumor has infiltrated the orbital roof, i.e., anterior cranial fossa, the ethmoid and frontal sinus and dura, it shall be removed in block along with all the affected structures [15, 24, 31] (Figure 16). On the basis of correct diagnosis this should be anticipated preoperatively. In such cases, after coronal incision, the dissection of the soft tissues is performed in a subfolicular, i.e., supragaleal layer. After reaching the supraorbital region, it is necessary to enter into the subperiosteal level in order to explore the orbit and preserve the supraorbital and the supratrochlear neurovascular bundle. Then the galea with periost is lifted as a separate flap based on the temporal blood vessels (Figure 12). Before returning the bone fragments this flap is placed onto the base of the brain or into the frontal sinus, in which previously cranialisation is performed, in order to separate dura and brain from the nasal cavum. Separation of dura and brain from the nasal cavum, i.e., prevention of meningitis and encephalitis, can only be done by a living tissue, i.e., by a vascularized flap.

The superior and the lateral part of the orbit can be reached by various transcranial, neurosurgical approaches [31, 33], by using various methods of removal of the roof and the lateral orbital wall (Figure 13).

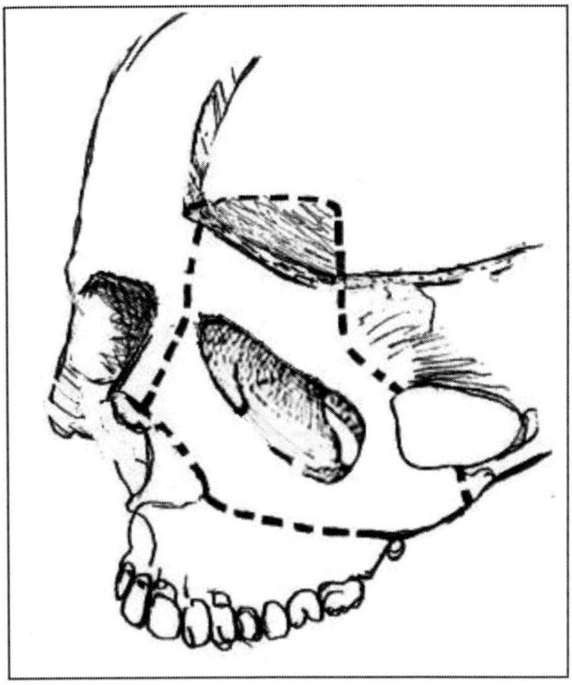

Figure 14. A drawing of a removal of facial skeleton and the tumor of the orbit.

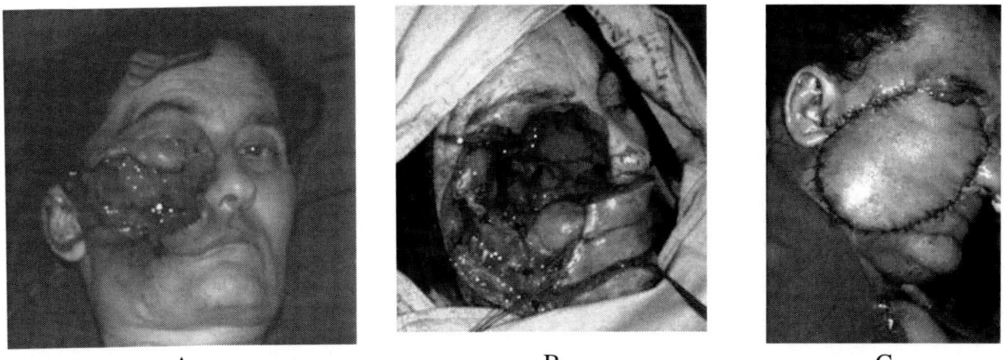

A B C

Figure 15. A. The facial tumor that has spread onto the orbit. B. The tumor has been removed along with the orbit, its content, frontal sinus and the part of the skull base. C. The defect has been covered by a pectoral musculocutaneous flap, which has been transferred on the pedicle of the acromiopectoral artery and vein.

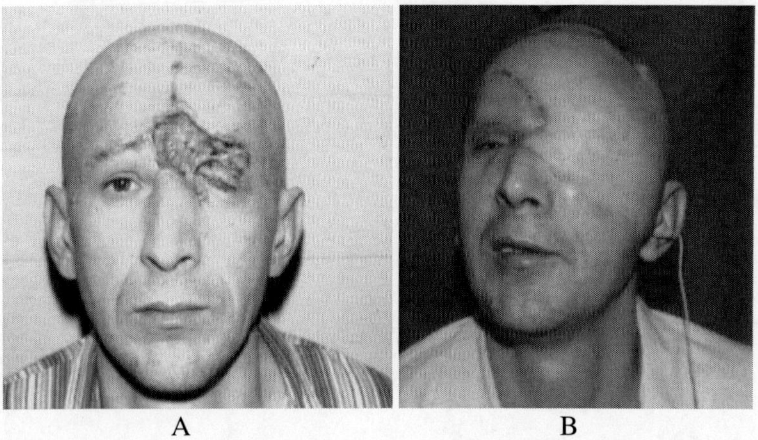

Figure 16. A. The patient with a basocellular carcinoma of the frontoethmoid region and the orbit. B. Together with the tumor, part of the frontal bone, part of the frontal brain lobe, the ethmoid and the frontal sinus, the anterior part of the skull base and the orbit have also been removed in block. The deformity has been covered by latissimus dorsi musculocutaneous flap, which has been transferred by a microsurgical vascular anastomosis.

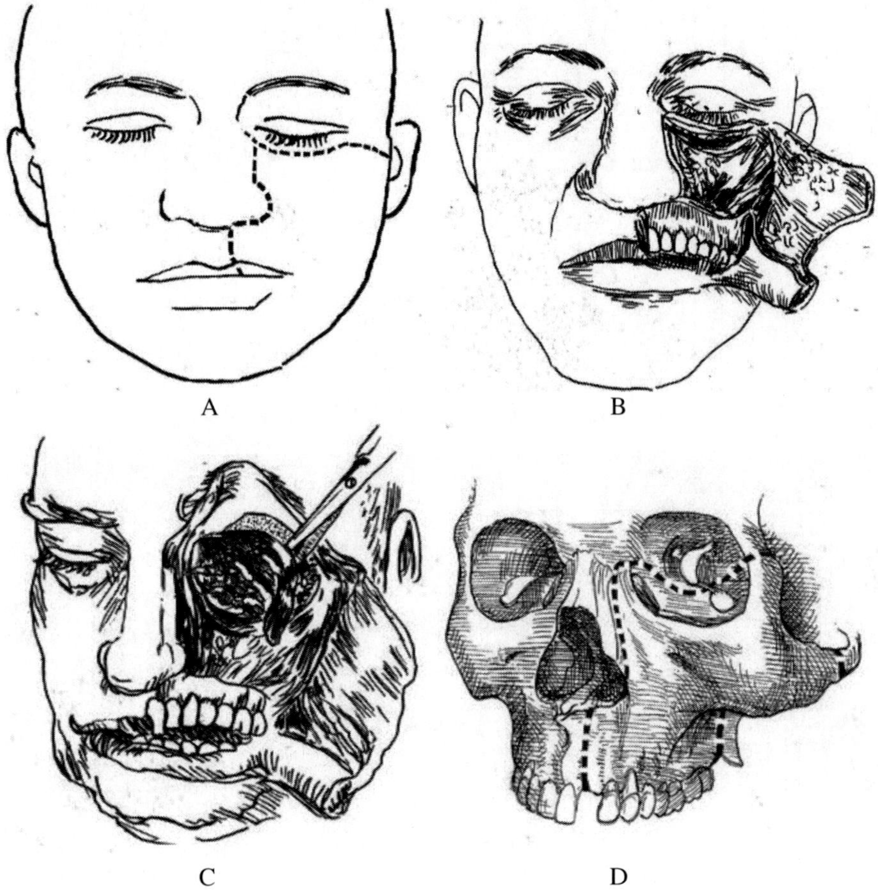

Figure 17. A, B, C, D. Weber-Ferguson approach for radical resection of the maxilla and exenteration of the orbit.

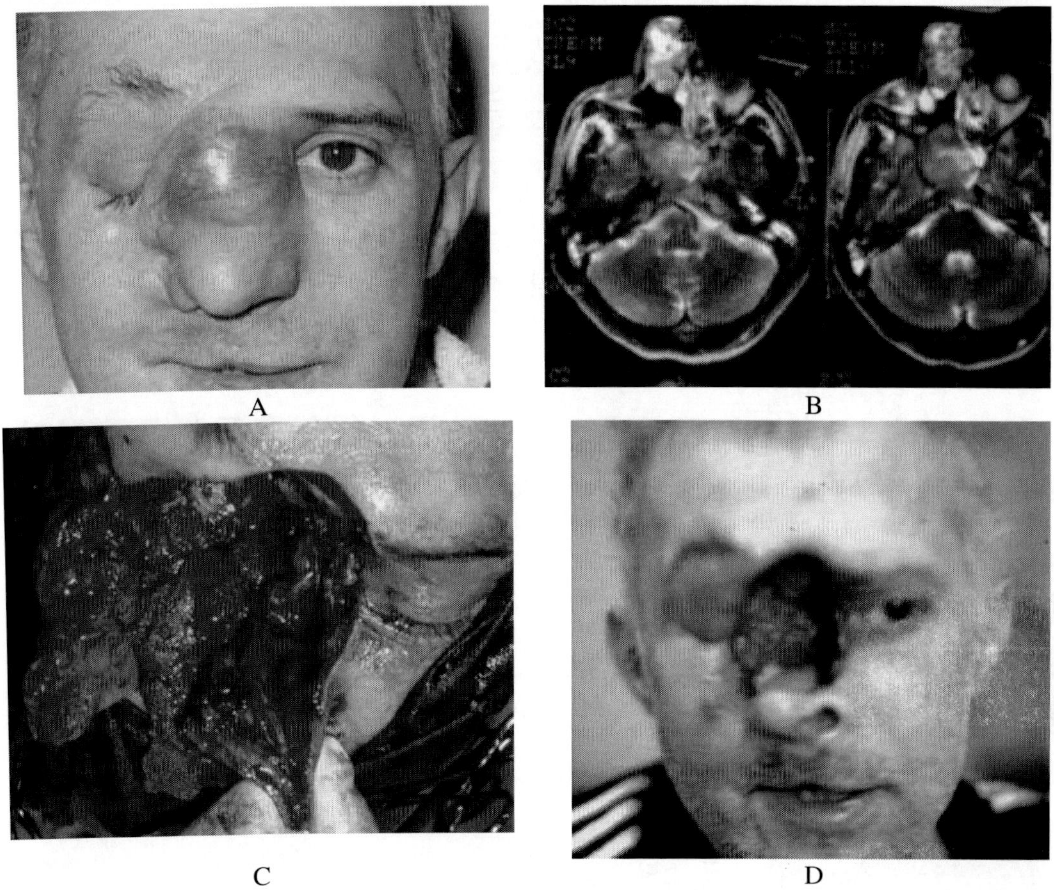

Figure 18. A, B. The tumor of the nasoethmoid region and the cranial base that has penetrated the orbit. C. The tumor has been removed with exenteration of the orbit, together with the medial part of the orbit. D. The condition one month after the operation. The patient has been prepared for the construction of episthesis.

In cases of extensive pathological lesions of the facial skeleton, the paranasal sinuses and the cranial base, which also affect the orbit, the orbit can be reached by various complicated transfacial approaches [33], which is in the domain of craniofacial surgery. In such cases, the orbit, or part of orbit, is also removed along with the tumor, with or without exenteration (Figures 14, 15, 16, 17, 18). In case of the malignant tumor of the maxilla or the maxillary sinus that has penetrated the orbit, most often, by using a Weber-Ferguson approach, the exenteration of the orbit must be performed along with the maxilla removal (Figure 17).

When a tumor from the nose and the ethmoid sinus penetrates the orbit, the medial part of the orbit shall also be removed along with tumor, with or without exenteration (Figure 18). The tumors of the retro-maxillary space (Figure19) and of the cranial base (Figure 20) can also penetrate the orbit. Using a transfacial approach - a temporary separation of the facial bones from the skull – by osteotomy of the facial skeleton according to the type Le Fort II or Le Fort III (Figure 20) or by some other similar approach (Figure 19) the tumor can be reached. Together with the tumor a part of the orbit shall be also removed, with or without exenteration. After the tumor removal the facial skeleton shall be returned to its original position and fixed by a stainless steel wire 0.4 mm thick or by mini i.e., micro plates.

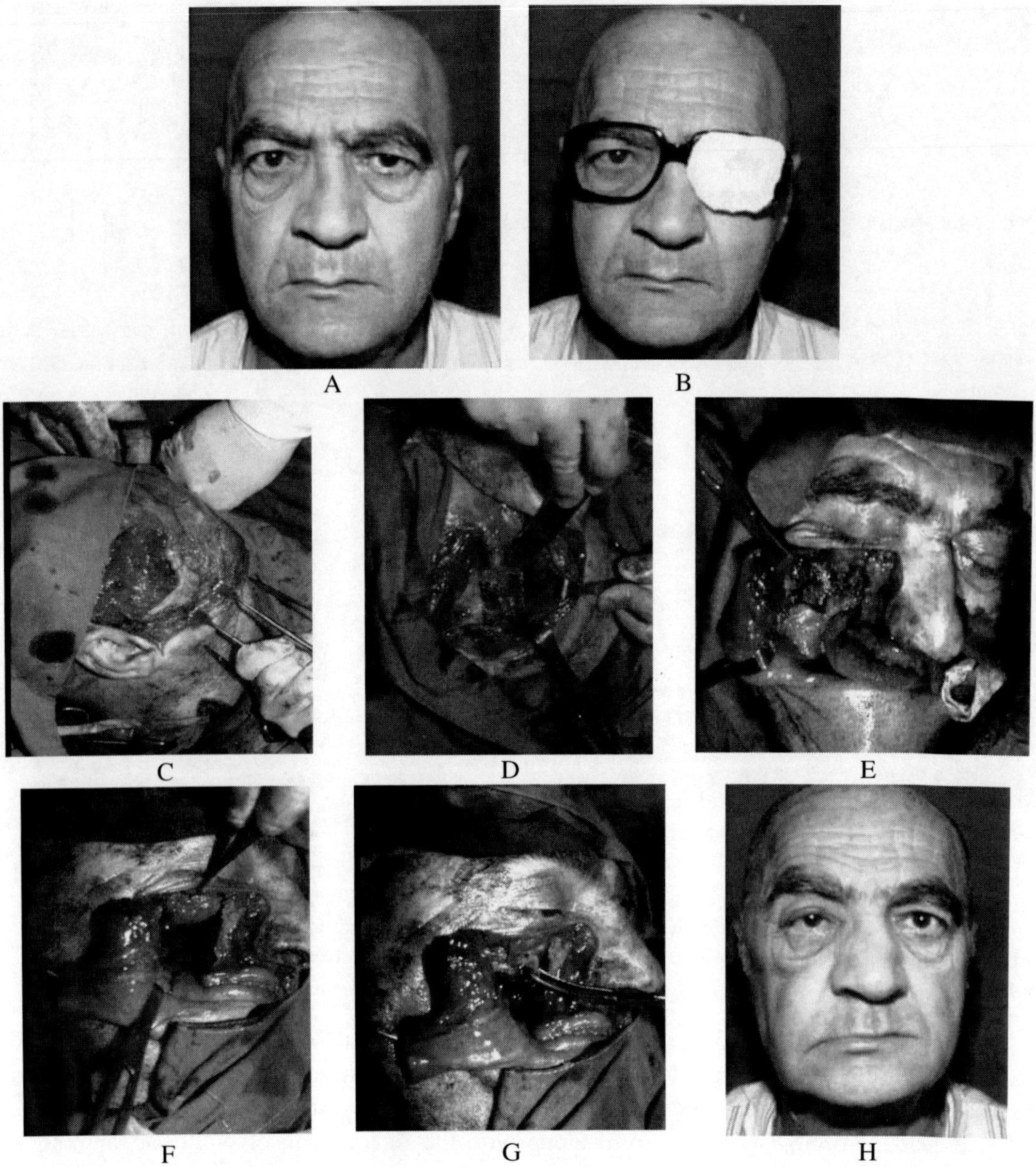

Figure 19. A. The patient with the tumor of the retromaxillary space and the right eye protrusion. B. Because of the double vision the patient has a mask on one side of the glasses. C. The zygomatic arch is reached by a coronal approach. D. The zygomatic arch has been temporarily removed and the tumor in the retromaxilalry space is approached through the infratemporal fossa. E. By applying the Weber-Ferguson approach, the anterior part of the maxilla has been osteotomized and moved to the side together with the soft tissues so the tumor in retromaxillary space is reached from the maxillary side. F. The tumor has been removed together with a part of the cranial base and the orbital floor. The eyeball hangs in empty space. G. Reconstruction of the orbital floor has been performed by a coronoid process of the mandible, which has been transferred on the temporal muscle. H. The zygomatic arch and the anterior part of the maxilla have been returned to their original position and fixed by wire ligatures. Soft tissues have been returned to their positions. The right eye has a good position and there is no double vision.

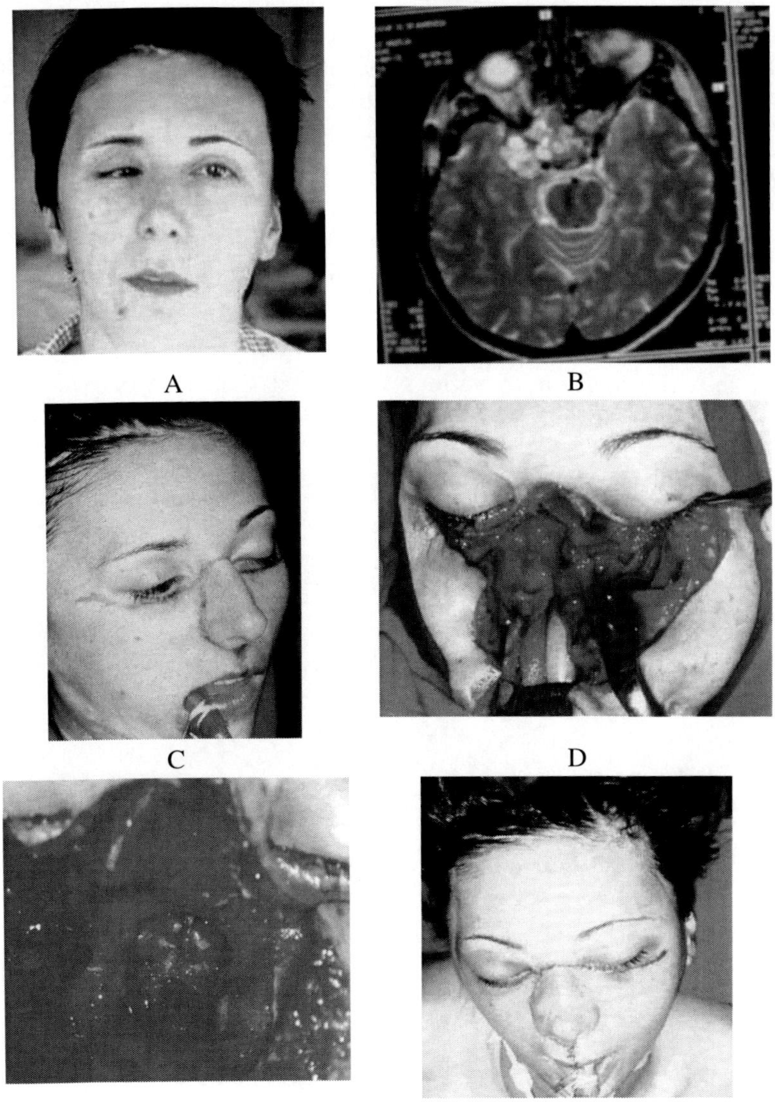

Figure 20. A. B. The patient with a cranial base tumor that has penetrated into the apical part of the right orbit. Vision is lost in the right eye due to the optic nerve compression. III, V and VI nerve have been damaged. In the previous two operations the tumor has not been removed. During the first operation, in neurosurgical hospital, it was impossible to reach the tumor by using a neurosurgical transcranial approach. During the second operation, in the same hospital, a part of the maxilla and the orbital floor have been removed through the maxillary sinus, with the tumor biopsy. Due to removal of the orbital floor the patient has enophthalmos. C. The drawing of incision for a bilateral transfacial approach to the cranial base tumor that has penetrated the orbit. D. Bilaterally performed Le Fort III osteotomy of the facial bones. The facial bones have been separated from the cranial bones and moved downwards. The osteotomy is performed in the medial line, and the middle third of the face is separated. On the right side there are the maxilla and the zygomatic bone with the remnants of the right orbital floor, and on the left – the nose, the maxilla and the zygomatic bone with the left orbital floor. E. The tumor has been removed. F. The facial bones have been returned to their original position and fixed by mini plates. The osteoplastiy of the right orbital floor has been performed by using a piece of the calvarial bone.

3.5.3.4. Exenteration of the Orbit

The exenteration of the orbit represents a surgical procedure that implies the removal of the eye with the soft orbital structures, i.e., the removal of the eyelids, the extrabulbar muscles, the orbital fat tissue, the optic nerve and the periorbit [19, 23] (Figures 21, 22). The most common reason for exenteration of the orbit is advanced primary malignant (Figure 21) and secondary malignant (Figure 22) orbital tumor. Exenteration of the orbit has also been indicated in cases of meningioma, neurofibromatosis, hemangioma, lymphangioma and similar pathological processes that have caused major orbital deformations, with pain and loss of vision. In cases of dangerous (fungal) infections affecting the orbit and the paranasal sinuses, particularly in diabetics and people with weakened immunity, in addition to exenteration of the orbit and due to various reasons, it shall also be necessary to perform debridement of the paranasal sinuses, and sometimes of the adjacent cranial fossa.

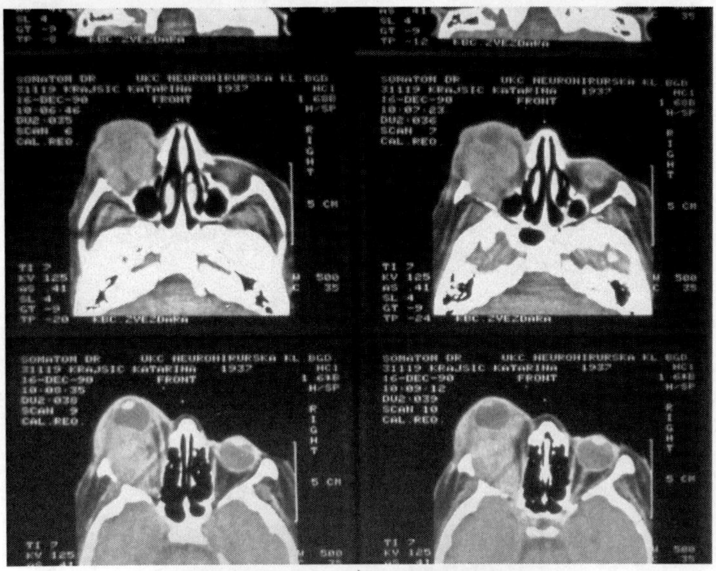

A

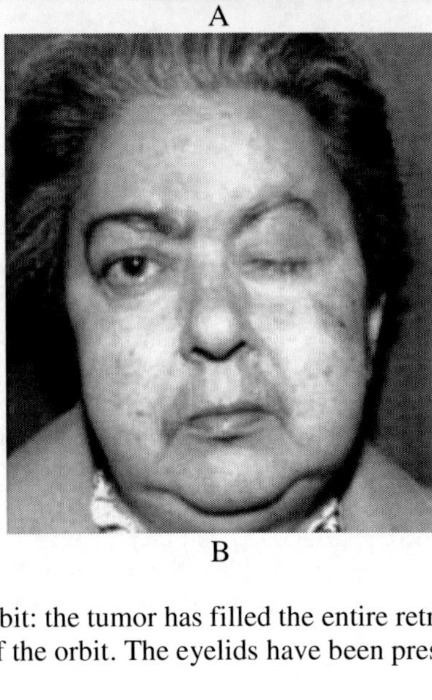

B

Figure 21. A. CT image of the orbit: the tumor has filled the entire retrobulbar space of the orbit. B. The same patient after exenteration of the orbit. The eyelids have been preserved.

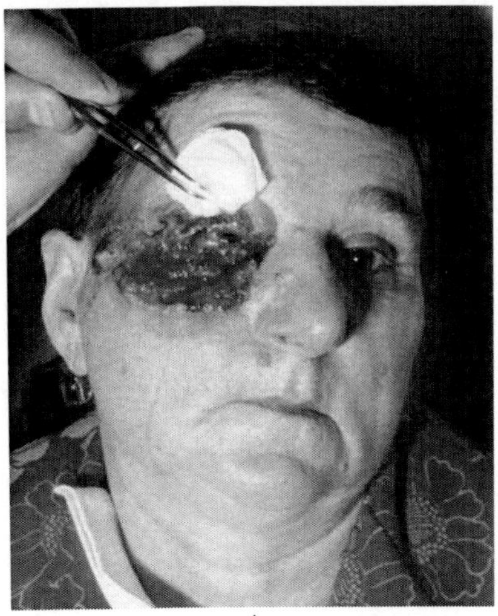

A

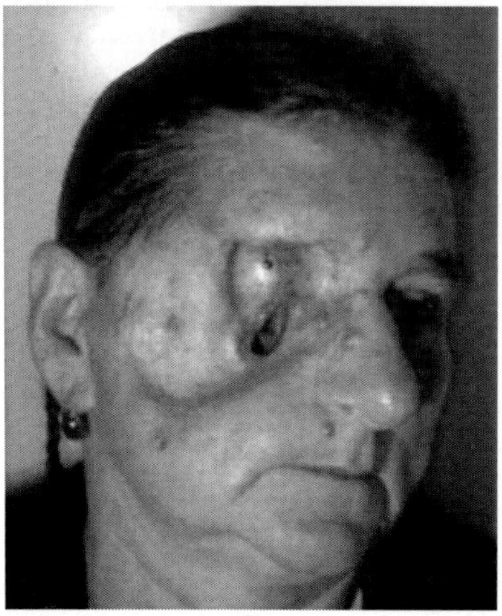

B

Figure 22. A. The eyelid carcinoma that has spread onto the facial bones and the orbit *per continuitatem*. B. A larger part of the maxilla, zygomatic bone and the orbit have been removed, with exenteration of the orbit. The wound has been covered by a free split thickness skin graft.

The surgery starts with the incision to the eyelids. The incision is made deep to the bone and must be at a sufficient distance from the tumor edge (for malignant tumors this should be no less than 1 cm). Once the bone has been reached, periosteum is cut by a scalpel, and then the entire inner surface of the orbit, to the apex, is being deperiosted. In this way, the orbital content shall be separated from the orbital walls. In the area of the orbital apex, i.e., in the area of the optic nerve and the ophthalmic artery, hemostatic forceps is inserted and the tissue is cut by a knife or scissors. It is necessary to put a stronger ligature at the cutpoint. If the pathological process has spread onto some of the orbital walls or has penetrated the paranasal sinuses, then both the orbital wall and the affected part of the sinus shall be removed in block with the orbital structures (Figures 14-22). After such operations the orbital wound can be covered in various ways. The simplest method is to "pack" the orbit by a gauze impregnated with iodoform or antibiotic ointment and, with regular cleaning and bandaging, wait for the granulations which will cover the orbital cavity [23]. Within 6 – 8 weeks epithelium is formed over the granulations. This period can be reduced if a free split thickness skin graft is placed over the granulations (Figure 22). In the course of operation it is possible to lift the pericranial galeoperiostal flap, based on the temporal blood vessels (Figure 12), and by this flap cover the orbital cavity. If this is done, the split thicknees skin graft is placed over the flap. The galeoperiostal flap can be placed into the orbit over the lateral margin or through the lateral wall, on which an opening has been formed by removing the bone. Through the opening on the lateral orbital wall it is possible to pull the temporal muscle into the orbit. If this is done, it is necessary to cover the muscle by free split thickness skin graft.

The orbital cavity can also be covered by various local or distant cutaneous or musculocutaneous flaps (Figure 15), and by diverse flaps transferred by microsurgical anastomosis of the blood vessels (Figure 16). The covering of the orbital cavity by various flaps has also a disadvantage, i.e., an inability to diagnose an early tumor recurrence.

After the completion of comprehensive therapy – a surgical one, that has been supplemented with irradiation therapy, and sometimes by polychemotherapy, and after confirmation that there is no recurrence, a patient can be subject to various reconstructive surgical or prosthetic procedures [8]. If it is possible to reconstruct the orbit, the eyelids and the conjunctival sacus, eye prosthesis is placed into the orbital cavity. A part of the orbit or the entire one, the eyelids and the eye can be created as a prosthesis (episthesis) and fixed to glasses or the surrounding bones by osteointegrating metal implants which are drilled into the adjacent bone as pegs.

3.6. Patients and Surgical Therapy Results

Ninety-two people suffering from different types of orbital tumors were subject to different surgical procedures (Figures 1-22). In 17 cases when the tumor was located in the anterior half of the orbit, it was approached by anterior orbitotomy (Figures 1-6). In order to provide a better view, better approach to the tumor and reduced risk of damaging important structures in the orbit, a temporary marginectomy of the superior, inferior or lateral orbital margin was performed in 8 people (Figures 4, 6). In nine cases, when the tumor was located in the lateral part of the orbit, it was approached by the lateral orbitotomy (Figure 7, 8, 9). In 10 cases, when the tumor was found in the superior retrobulbar space of the orbit, it was necessary to perform a transcranial supraorbital orbitotomy in order to approach the tumor (Figures 10, 11, 12).

Due to the advanced malignant tumors of the eyelids and/or conjunctiva, mostly basocellular and squamocellular carcinoma, that have penetrated the orbit, thirty patients were subject to exenteration of the orbit (Figures 21, 22). In 26 people with advanced malignant tumors (paranasal sinuses, maxilla, retromaxillary space, the anterior region and the cranial base) which penetrated the orbit, the tumor has been removed in block with the entire orbit, or part of the orbit, with or without exenteration, by using various transfacial approaches (Figures 14 – 22). These procedures allow a wide approach to the orbit, and its direct inspection, which has considerably reduced the incidence of iatrogenic injuries of the orbital structures.

Conclusion

Surgical therapy is certainly the most effective method for orbital tumors. Taking orbital anatomy into consideration, along with functionality, and the topographic relations with the adjacent regions, orbital tumor surgery is very complex and requires mastering surgery of the surrounding regions, and quite frequently multidisciplinary teamwork. Thanks to the new advances in surgery, i.e., new transcranial and transfacial approaches, a better approach to orbital tumors has been provided. This has increased efficiency of surgical procedures and protection of the important orbital structures against iatrogenic injuries.

References

[1] Alper M. G., Bray M., Evaluation of a primary lymphoma of the orbit, *Br. J. Ophthalmol.*68: 255-260, 1984.

[2] Astaria R., Minckler D., Taylor C, Orbital and adnexal lymphomas, *Am. J. Clin. Pathol.*73: 615-621, 1980.

[3] Bech K., Jensen O. A., External ocular tumors, Georg Thieme, Stutgart, 1978.

[4] Berke R.N., A modified Kronlein operation, *Arch. Ophthalmol.*51: 609-632, 1954.

[5] Char D. H., Clinical ocular oncology, Churchill Livingstone, New York, Edinburgh, London, Melbourne, 1989.

[6] Chavis R. M., Gamer A., Wright J.E., Inflamatory orbital pseudotumor, *Arch. Ophthalmol.*96: 1817-1822, 1978.

[7] Conley J., The risk to the orbit in head and neck cancer, *Laryngoscope* 95: 515-522, 1985.

[8] De Breo E. L., Schiler D.E., Surgical and prosthetic consideration in the management of orbital tumors, *J. Prosth. Dent.*67: 106-112, 1992.

[9] Delashow J. B., Persing J.A., Lessner A. Supraorbital rim craniotomy and its variations, in: Toth B.A., Keating R.F., Stewart W.B., An atlas of orbitocranial surgery, Martin Dunitz, London, 1999.

[10] Font R.L., Ferry A.P., Carcinoma metastatic to the eye and orbit, *Cancer* 38: 1326 – 1335, 1978.

[11] Goldberg R. A., Anterior orbitotomy, in: Toth B. A., Keating R. F., Stewart W. B., An atlas of orbitocranial surgery, Martin Dunitz, London, 1999.

[12] Goldberg R. A., Rootman J., Clinical characteristics of methastatic orbital tumors, *Ophthalmology* 97: 620-524, 1990.

[13] Hi C., Abert D. M., Tumors of the eyelid and orbit: a Chinese – American collaborative study, *Int. Ophthalm. Clin.* 22: 1-5, 1982.

[14] Hornblass A., *Tumors of the ocular adnexa and orbit*, Mosby, St. Louis, 1979.

[15] Jackson I. T., Munro I. R., Sayler K. E., Whitaker L.A., *Atlas of Craniomaxillofacial Surgery*, Mosby, St. Louis, 1982.

[16] Knowless D. M., Jakobiec F. A., Orbital lymphoid neoplasms: A clinicopathologic study of 60 cases, *Cancer* 46: 576-589, 1980.

[17] Latković Z., Tumors of the eyelids, in: Litričin and al. Eye Tumors, Institute for Publishing Textboks and Teaching Materials, Belgrade, 1988.

[18] Lemke B. N., Della Rocca R. C., Surgery of the eyelid & orbits, Prentice-Hall International Inc., 1990.

[19] Levin P. S., Toth B.A., Orbital exenteration in: Toth B. A., Keating R. F., Stewart W. B., *An atlas of orbitocranial surgery*, Martin Dunitz, London, 1999.

[20] Litričin O., *Tumors of the orbit*, in: Litričin and al. Eye Tumors, Institute for Publishing Textboks and Teaching Materials, Belgrade, 1988.

[21] Maroon J.C., Kennerdell J.S., Surgical approaches to the orbit: indications and techniques, *J. Neurosurg*. 60: 1226-1235, 1984.

[22] Mohr C., Schettler D., Heesen J., The surgical approach to orbital space-occupying lesions, *J. Cranio-Max.-Fac. Surg*.17:149-154, 1989.

[23] Putterman A.M., Orbital exenteration with spontaneous granulation, *Arch. Ophthalmol.*104: 139-140, 1986.

[24] Raveh J., Vuillemin T., Subcranial-supraorbital and temporal approach for tumor resection, *J.Craniofac.Surg*. 1: 53-59, 1990.

[25] Reese A.B., *Tumors of the eye*, Hoeber, New York, 1951.

[26] Rončević R., Fibrous displasia of facial and skull bones, Serbian Archive 113: 63-70, 1985.

[27] Rončević R., Modern concepts of the treatment and prognosis of malignant skin tumors, *Serbian Archive* 122: 358-363, 1994.

[28] Rončević R., Osvald M., Popović M., Potentials of X-ray diagnostics in maxillofacial region, *Chirurgia Maxillofac.-plastica* 11: 47-54, 1980.

[29] Sesenna E., Raffaini M., Tullio A., Moscato G., Orbital marginotomies for treatment of orbital and periorbital lesions, *Int. J. Oral. Maxillofac. Surg*. 23: 76-84, 1994.

[30] Shields J. A., Bakewell B., Classification and incidence of space-occupying lesions of the orbit. A survey of 645 biopsies, *Arch. Ophthalmol* 102: 1606-1611, 1984.

[31] Stewart W. B., Toht B. A., A multidisciplinary approach to orbital neoplasm *Clin. Plast Surg*. 15: 263-272, 1988.

[32] Sullivan W. G., Kawamoto H. K., Periorbital margionotomies: anatomy and applications, *J. Cranio-Max.-Fac. Surg*. 17: 206-209, 1989.

[33] Toth. B. A., Keating R. F., Stewart W. B., *An atlas of orbitocranial surgery,* Martin Dunitz, London, 1999.

[34] Zimmerman L. E., Sobin L. H., Histological typing of tumours of the eye and adnexa, internat. *Histological classification of tumours*, No 24, WHO, Geneva, 1980.

Chapter 4

Surgical Treatment of Dysthyroid Ophthalmopathy

4.1. Introduction

Disorders of the thyroid gland are manifested by numerous symptoms, such as restlessness, anxiety, tremor, tachycardia, fatigue, perspiration, hyperexcitability of the digestive tract, weight loss, and various changes in the eyes and the eye adnexa. Back in 1786, Caleb Parry first noticed bulging eyes in a patient suffering from the thyroid gland disorder and he published the finding in 1825. In 1835 Robert Graves [11] described three patients who, in addition to the thyroid gland dysfunction, also had exophthalmos. In 1840 von Basedow published the precise data about the exophthalmos in patients diagnosed with hyperthyroidism. From this first written data about thyroid exophthalmos, to the present, a tremendous amount of information about this disease has been discovered, but even still much remains unknown. Even the name of this disease has not been agreed upon to this day. A great number of names are being used, such as Graves' ophthalmopathy, Graves' orbitopathy, Graves-Basedow's ophthalmopathy or orbitopathy, endocrine ophthalmopathy or orbitopathy, endocrine exophthalmos, thyroid, thyrotoxic or dysthyroid exophthalmos, thyroid or dysthyroid ophthalmopathy or orbitopathy, thyroid eye disease, immunogenic ophthalmopathy etc. None of these names is quite precise. Since the orbits, i.e., bone was not affected by a pathological process, but only the contents of the orbit, it seems that ophthalmopathy is more accurate a name than orbitopathy, especially as the organ of vision, in the wider sense of the word, consists of the eyeball and accessory organs of the eye (eyelids, eye muscles, lacrimal apparatus and orbital adipose tissue). Although today the most often used term is Graves' ophthalmopathy, the title of this chapter uses the term dysthyroid ophthalmopathy as a dysfunction of the thyroid gland is probably the "trigger" for this pathological condition. Today the name thyroid exophthalmos is rarely in use, although exophthalmos is the main symptom of this disease.

4.2. Etiopathogenesis of Dysthyroid Ophthalmopathy

Etiopathogenesis of Graves-Basedow disease is still not explained. Even less clear is the etiopathogenesis of Graves-Basedow ophthalmopathy, endocrine ophthalmopathy, dysthyroid ophthalmopathy. We are not yet sure whether the functional impairment of the thyroid gland and of the eyes and eye sockets content are one or two adjacent diseases. We are also not sure which dysfunction of the thyroid gland is a cause or "trigger" for development of dysthyroid ophthalmopathy. With regard to etiopathogenesis of dysthyroid ophthalmopathy, many attitudes are hypothetical, controversial and at the level of speculation even today. Changes in the eyes and the orbital content may occur in patients with hyperthyroidism, but also in euthyroid or hypothyroid individuals.

Wiersinga [40] gives the following facts: in 77% of the patients dysthyroid ophthalmopathy occurs together with hyperthyroidism, in 21% of the cases it occurs in euthyroid people, and 2% of the patients were diagnosed with hypothyroidism. Over twenty years Karageorgos et al. [15] studied 155 patients with dysthyroid ophthalmopathy. One hundred and thirty of them had hyperthyroidism, 15 were euthyroid, whereas 10 patients had hypothyroidism. The level of thyroid hormones, thyreo-stimulative hormone, and the severity of hyperthyroidism often do not correlate with the degree and severity of ophthalmopathy, and according to some researches they do not have any direct effect on the changes on the eyes and the eye adnexa. In patients in which the dysthyroid ophthalmopathy is associated with hyperthyreoidism, treatment of hyperthyroidsm may cause aggravation of the ophthalmopathy condition. Karageorgos et al. [15] specify that aggravation of the ophthalmopathy occurred in 14% of the patients treated with carbimazole, in 17% treated with radioactive iodine and in 12% after thyroidectomy.

Beside a nubmer of hypotheses and theories about etiopathogenesis of the dysthyroid ophthalmopathy, the prevailing opinion nowadays is that this is an autoimmune multifactorial process.[5, 7, 12, 18, 20, 40, 41]. The most often stressed fact is that the activated T-cells against antigenes of the folicular cells of the thyroid gland recognize similar antigenes in the orbital tissue and attach to those. These activated orbital T-cells release various cytokines that stimulate the production of glycosaminoglycane and colagen from the orbital fibroblasts, which causes inflammatory and oedematous changes in the orbit [5].

Numerous papers on the autoimmune pathogenesis and pathophysiology of the dysthyroid ophthalmopathy are in many ways speculative and controversial. Controversial are the facts about what is primary in the autoimmune process, who is responsible for common antigenes in the orbit and the thyroid gland, then about the function of the circulating antibodies against the extraocular muslces and the fibroblast components etc. The following question could be also put forward: if the dysthyroid ophthalmopathy is an autoimmune disease, how then can it be explained, that the most efficient therapy for this disease is surgical therapy, i.e., abundant orbital decompression. Decompression does not eliminate the cause and the mechanism of the autoimmune process. If, along with decompression, the orbital fat tissue has been removed along with the removal of the orbital walls, it may have a double effect. The removal of the orbital fat tissue has the effect of additional decompression, and it is plausible that this is the tissue where the autoimmune processes are happening. It is also unclear why only 5% of people with hyperthyroidism have manifested changes in the eyes. Heritage, sex, age, and some external factors, like stress and smoking play a certain role in the occurrence of dysthyroid ophthalmopathy. Women have the disease much more frequently than men – approximately 4:1, whereas the clinical picture in men is more severe.

4.3. Clinical Picture of Dysthyroid Ophthalmopathy – Changes on the Eyes and the Eye Adnexa

Dysthyroid ophthalmopathy most often occurs in a less severe form, as a non-infiltrative ophthalmopathy, with insignificant infiltration of the orbital tissue. Infiltrative ophthalmopathy with marked infiltration of the orbital tissue and severe clinical picture is much more rare (Figures 2-18).

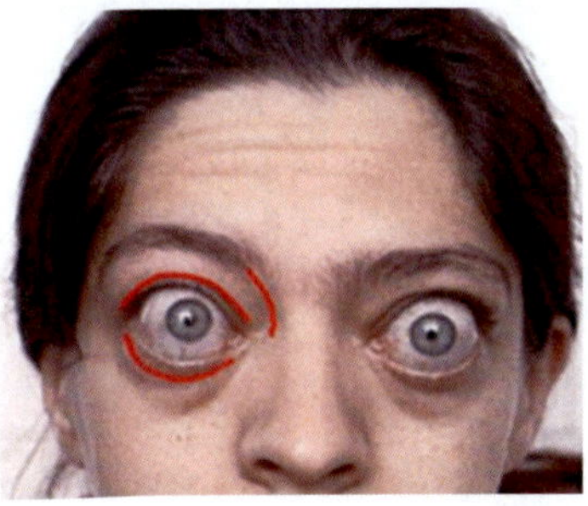

A

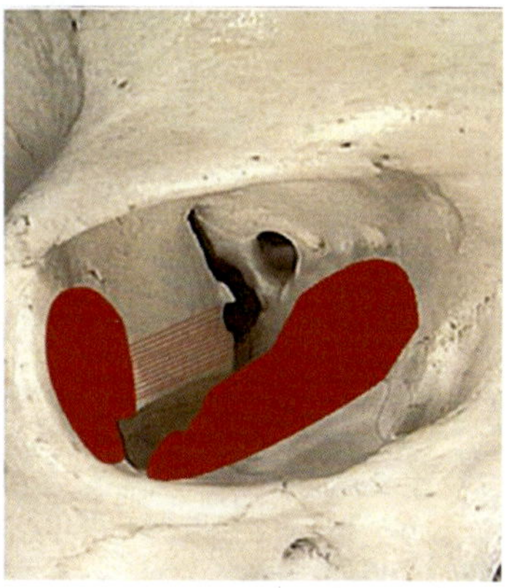

B

Figure 1. The approaches to the orbital walls are marked on the eyelids. The surgical bony defect is marked on the orbital walls.

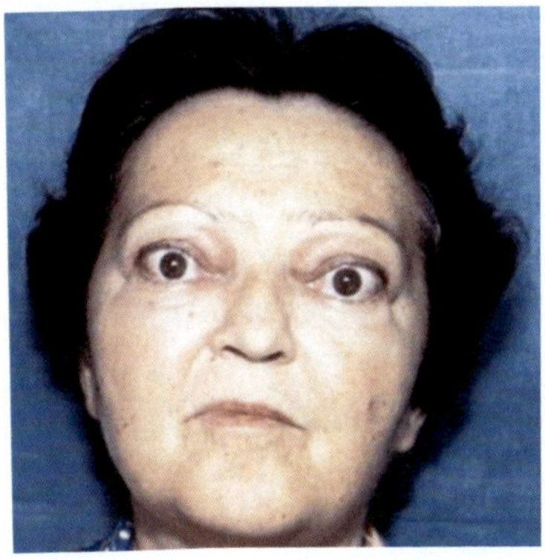

A

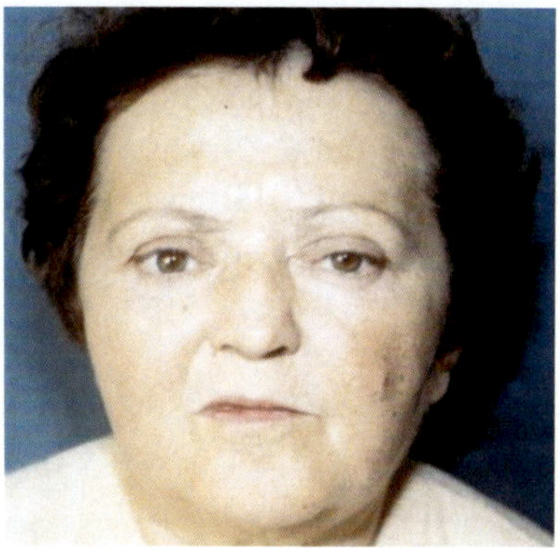

B

Figure 2. A. Patient with exophthalmos of 28 mm and eyelid deformities. B-3 months after the operation.

Table 1. Werner's classification of eye changes in patients suffering from dysthyroid ophthalmopathy

Class	Subclass	Gradation proposal
0		No physiological signs or symptomes
1		Only signs
 2	 o a b c	Changes on the soft tissues: Absence Minimum Medium Considerable
 3	 o a b c	Exophthalmos 3 mm or bigger: Absence From 3 to 4 mm beyond the upper limit of normal From 5 to 7 mm beyond the upper limit of normal 8 mm or more beyond the upper limit of normal
   4	 o a b c	Changes on the affected extraocular muscles (usually with diplopia): Absence Limited motility towards the ultimate borders of the gaze Obvious limitation of motility Fixation of the eyeball or the eyeballs
  5	 o a b c	Changes on the cornea (primarily due to lagophthalmos): Absence Spotty changes on the cornea Ulceration Blurred vision
  6	 o a b c	Weakening of the eyesight due to the affected optic nerve: Absence Pale or atrophic papilla or defects in the visual field, visual acuity from 20/20 to 20/60 Same, but visual acuity from 20/70 to 20/200 Blindness, i.e., decrease in light perception, visual acuity less than 20/200

Exophthalmos (proptosis) is the most frequent and the most significant manifestation of dysthyroid ophthalmopathy, but the degree of exophthalmos does not always correlate with the severity of disease and the severity of subjective difficulties. The degree of exophthalmos, and other changes as well, is often not the same in both eyes (Figures 3, 4, 5, 6, 7, 10) and sometimes the manifested disease occurs only in one eye (Figures 3,4) If the manifested disease is unilateral, it will most often start to develop in the other eye as well, possibly in a few months or maybe years.

The severity of the clinical picture of dysthyroid ophthalmopathy depends on the changes on the eyes and its adnexa. The severity of pathological changes is often not proportional in all structures, so various clinical forms can be seen. Due to all this, it is impossible to carry out a precise classification of the severity of this disease. Werner [39] classified the disease into six classes, by severity of the disease, i.e., by severity of the changes on the eyes and the eye adnexa, and each classe has been divided into several subclases (Table 1). It can be easily observed that in most of the patients with a severe form of dysthyroid ophthalmopaty there are changes characteristic for most or all classes.

Most patients have swollen eyelids, with significant retraction (Figures 2, 3, 4, 6, 11, 12, 13, 14, 15, 17, 18). The retraction of the upper eyelids is more significant and occurs mostly due to infiltration, fibrosis and adhesion of the upper eyelid levator muscle. However, retraction of the upper eyelid is also affected by increased tonus of the sympaticus which causes retraction of the Müller's muscle, as well as the exophthalmos itself. Similar processes also cause, although rarely, retraction of the lower eyelids. Deformity of the eyelids, apart from swelling, can be also caused by herniation of the orbital fat tissue, and also by swelling of the lacrimal gland protruding beyond the orbit.

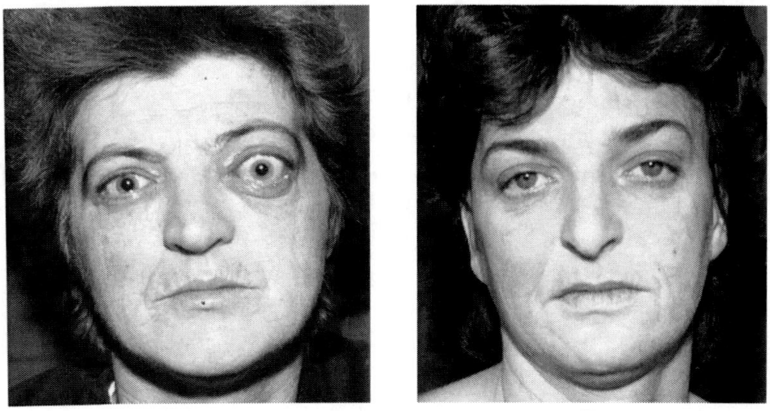

A B

Figure 3. A. Unilateral DO. B. One year after the operation.

The changes in the eyelids are manifested by various signs, which were named by the authors: retraction of the upper eyelids – Dalrymple's sign, lagging of the upper eyelids on downward gaze, rotation of the eye – Graefe's sign, rarely blinking – Stellwag's sign, increased retraction during fixation – Kocher's sign, and tremor of the eyelids when the eyes are closed – Rosenbach's sign.

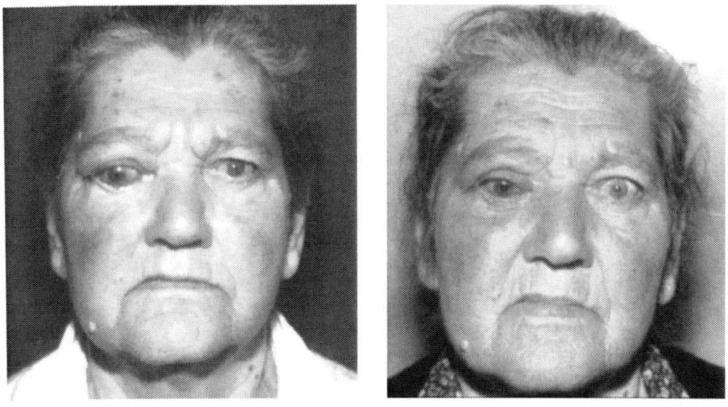

A B

Figure 4. A. Patient of 73 years with unilateral DO. B. 7 days after the operation.

Hyperemia of various degree or chemosis are most often developed on the conjunctiva. In the most severe cases conjunctiva prolapses over the eyelid rim, particularly the lower one (Figures 13, 17). These changes occur due to the vein congestion caused by the obstruction of the ophthalmic vein branches. This congestion pressures the lacrimal glands and ducts, which may cause decrease in lacrimation. If due to the specified processes the position of the lacrimal points changes, the epiphora appears.

Due to the exophthalmos, the eyelid retraction, infrequent blinking, interruption of the tear film, and due to the pressure of the swollen eyelid, various changes occur in the cornea. The damage to the corneal epithelium escalates into keratitis. Should the process persist, ulceration may develop and may progress into perforation of the cornea.

In cases of manifested ophthalmopathy, with a significant exophthalmos, the extraocular muscles are swollen, thickened, elongated and strained. In the later phase of the disease fibrosis of muscles occurs. These processes in the muscles result in deterioration of their function, due to which double vision occurs, often with strabismus. The changes in the muscles most often affect the inferior and the internal rectus muscle.

In about 5% of all patients suffering from dysthyroid ophthalmopathy, the optic neuropathy of various intensity also occurs, with diverse changes on the papilla of the optic nerve – from hyperemia and edema to atrophy [14, 32, 35, 37]. It is believed that the changes of the optic nerve occur because the swollen, thickened extraocular muscles and the fat tissue put a direct pressure on the optic nerve and the blood vessels feeding this nerve. The damage of the optic nerve may also be the result of its stretching in cases of a significant exophthalmos [6, 35].

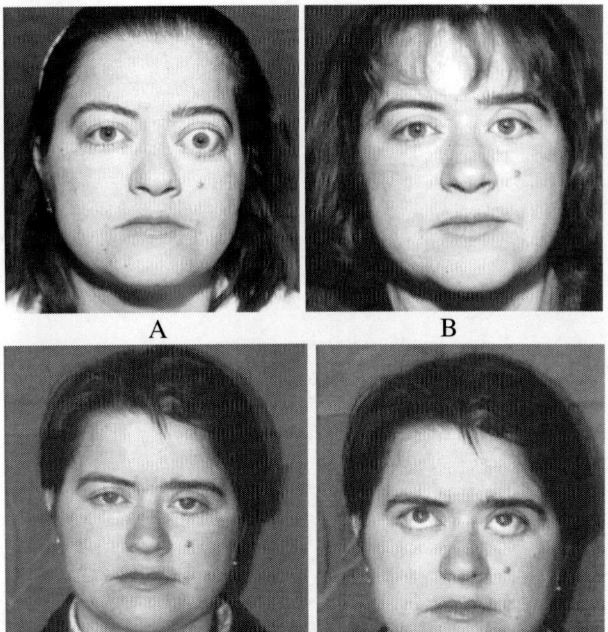

Figure 5. A. Patient with asymmetric exophthalmos. B. 3 months after the operation. C, D. 3 years after the operation.

There are various, even controversial data on the changes of the orbital fat tissue in patients suffering from dysthyroid ophthalmopathy. Most frequently it is stated that fat tissue volume has been increased due to infiltration with mucopolysaccharides, lymphocytes, macrophages, plasma cells and mast cells, and that thus enlarged fat tissue has an effect on the orbital pressure rise, and the occurrence of the exophthalmos [24, 40]. Often in the course of surgical procedures in severe cases of ophthalmopathy, the author of this book discovered degenerative and atrophic changes on the orbital fat tissue. Occasionally, in cases of the assymetric exophthalmos, due to the atrophic and degenerative changes of the fat tissue, the volume of this tissue was smaller on the side where the exophthalmos was more evident.

The exophthalmos, proptosis, protrusion of the eyeball is the most significant and the most noticeable manifestation of the dysthyroid ophthalmopathy. The regular values of the exophthalmos, i.e., the distance between the corneal apex and the external orbital margin differ among the races. The upper limit in Caucasians is 20 mm, in Mongolians it is 18 mm, and in Negroids about 22 mm. In females the upper limit is smaller by approximately 2 mm, and in children, it is proportional to their age. The size, i.e., the degree of exophthalmos is usually represented as displayed in the Table 2.

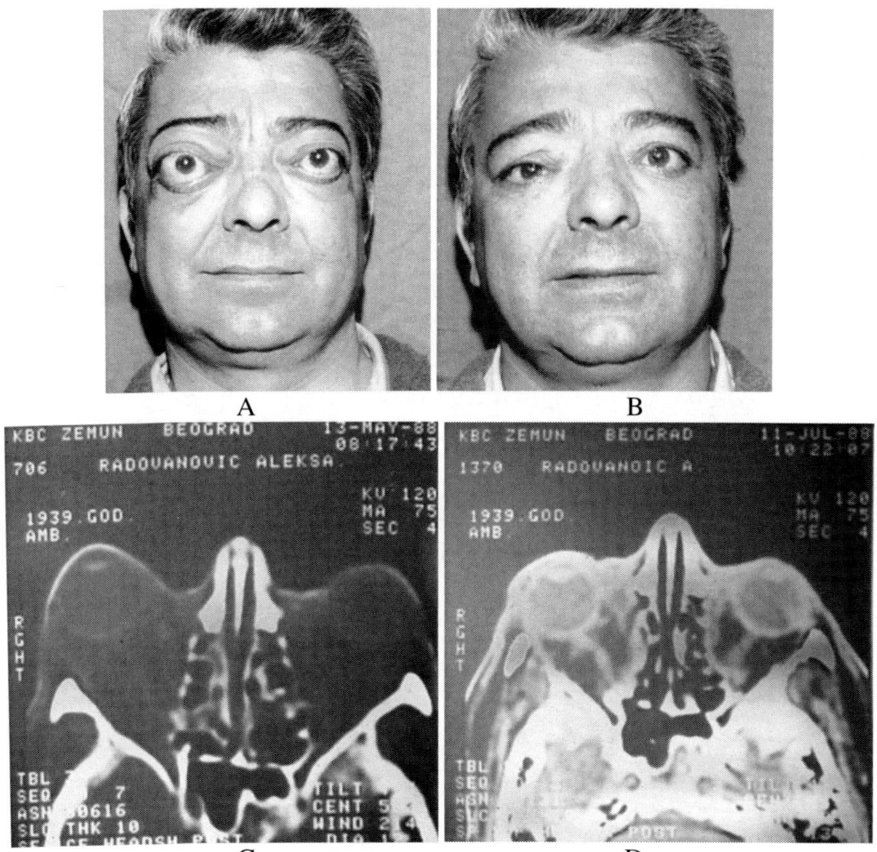

Figure 6. A. Patient with asymmetric exophthalmos of 32 mm and eyelid deformities. B. 2 months after the operation. C, D. CT of the same patient, before and 2 months after the operation.

What causes an occurrence of exophthalmos? – The increased orbital content due to the swelling and thickening of the extraocular muscles and the increase in volume of the orbital fat tissue and other tissues causes the rise of the orbital pressure, particularly in the narrow orbital apex. These enlarged tissues are not compressible, so therefore, a certain direction of their expansion is unavoidable. The exophthalmos would represent a spontaneous forward orbital decompression. The degree of exophthalmos does not always correlate with the severity of the disease, i.e., the severity of the symptoms (Figure 17). Some patients with very severe exophthalmos don't have serious difficulties, whereas others, with less evident exophthalmos may have severe ones. In some patients, mostly euthyroid ones, the exophthalmos is assymetrical or one-sided when the other eye is seemingly undamaged.

Table 2. Graduation of exophthalmos

DEGREE	SIZE (mm)
No exophthalmos	Up to 20 mm
Mild exophthalmos	21 -23 mm
Moderate exophthalmos	24 – 27 mm
Marked exophthalmos	Over 27 mm

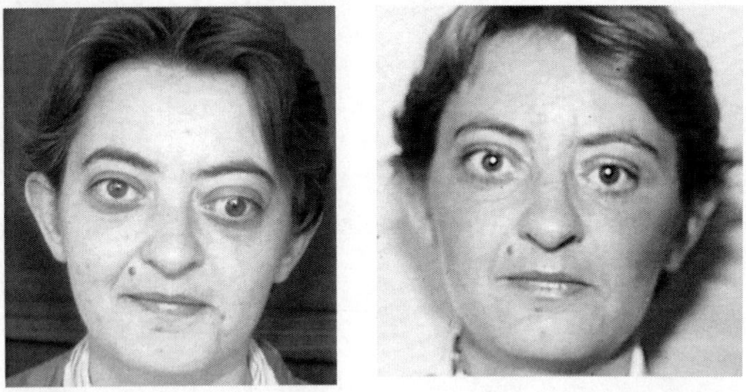

A B

Figure 7. A. Patient with exophthalmos of 28 mm and strabismus. B.3 months after operation.

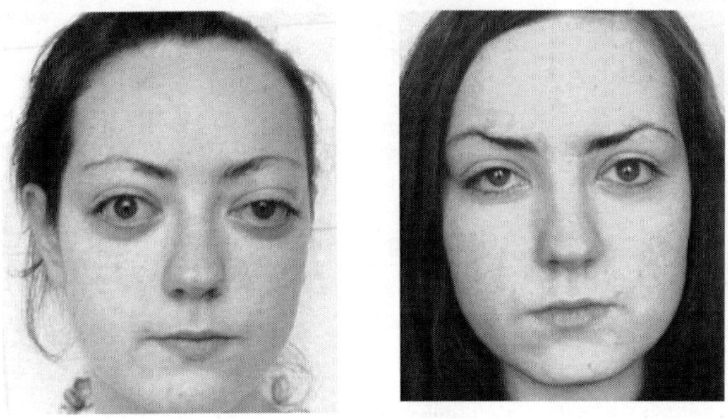

A B

Figure 8. A. Patient of 17 years after thyroidectomy with asymmetric exophthalmos and strabismus (changes on the eyes are worsened after thyroidectomy). B. 2 months after the operation.

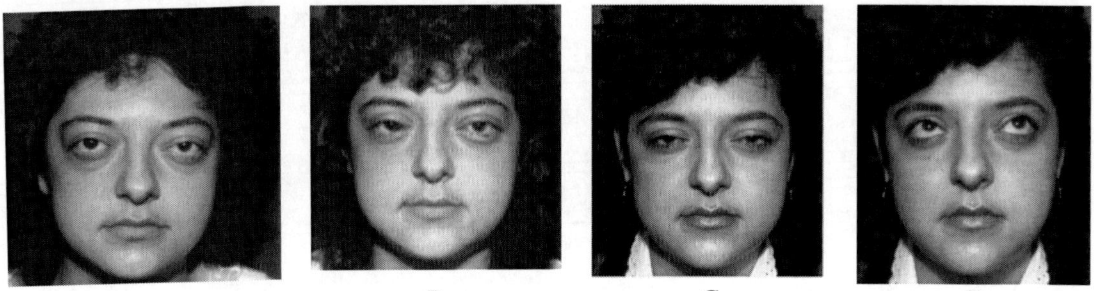

A B C D

Figure 9. A. Patient of 18 years with DO. B. 2 weeks after the operation. C, D - 2 years after the operation.

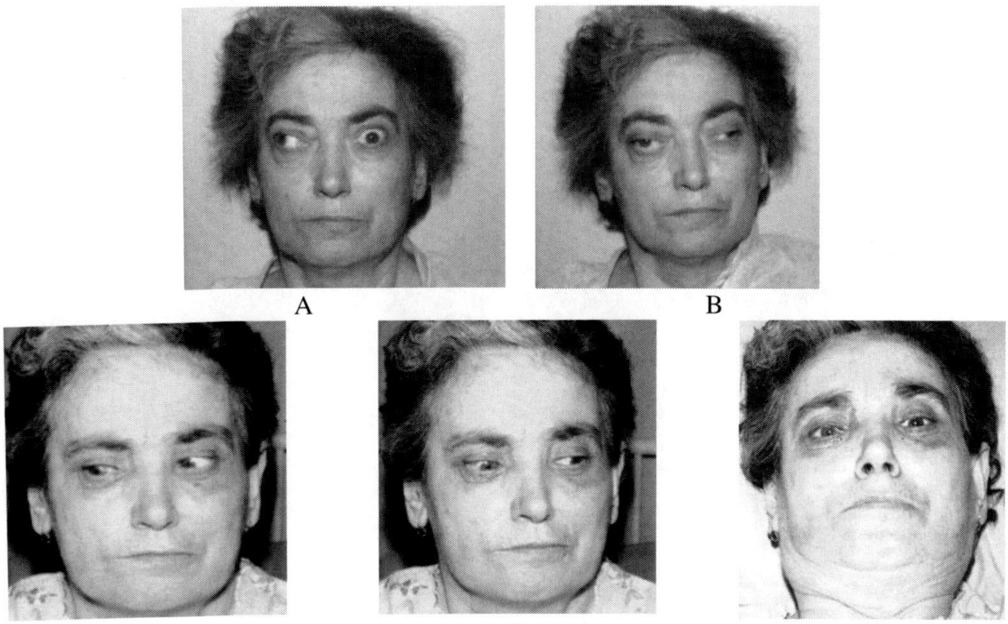

A B

C D E

Figure 10. A, B. Patient with asymmetric exophthalmos of 28 mm and strabismus. C, D, E. 11 days after the operation.

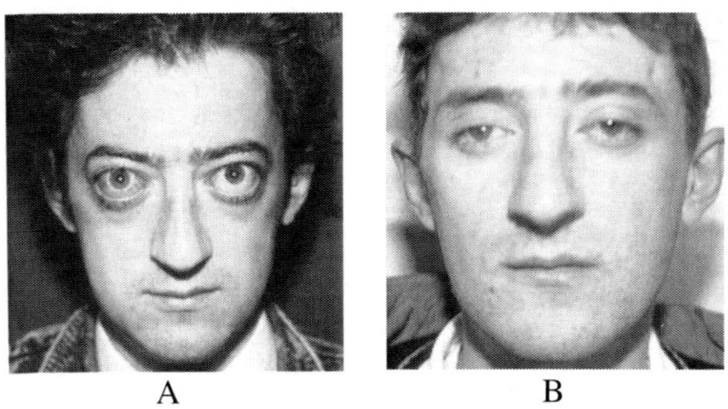

A B

Figure 11. A. Patient after Naffziger's neurosurgical orbital decompression (orbital roofs are removed) and radiation therapy with eyelid deformities, pulsatile exophthalmos of 30 mm and blindness on the right, before. B. 4 years after described orbital decompression and osteoplasty of the orbital roofs.

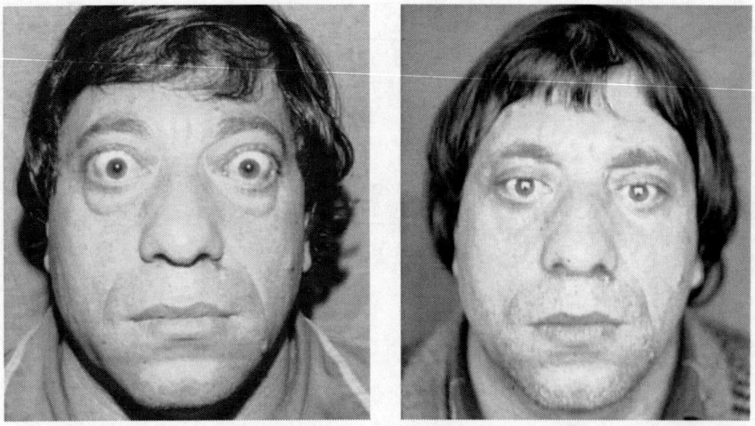

A B

Figure 12. A. Patient with exophthalmos of 30 mm and eyelid deformities. B. 3 month after the operation.

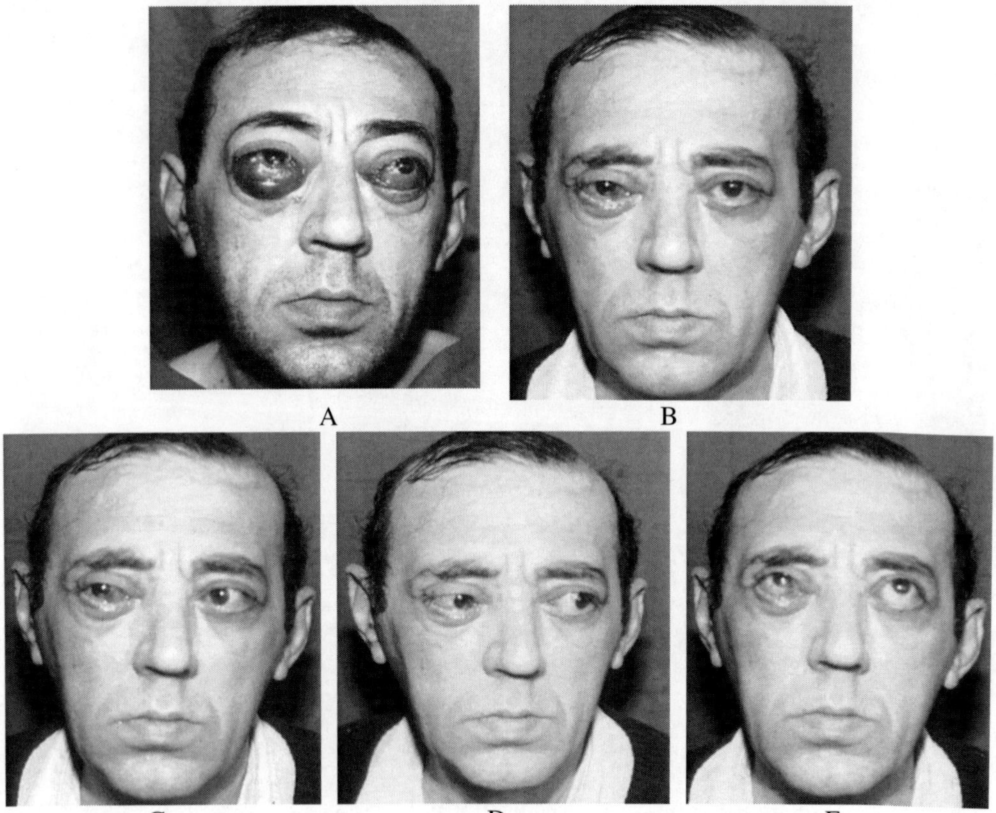

A B

C D E

Figure 13. A. Patient with malignant DO, exophtalmos of 33 mm. B, C, D, E. 3 weeks after the operation.

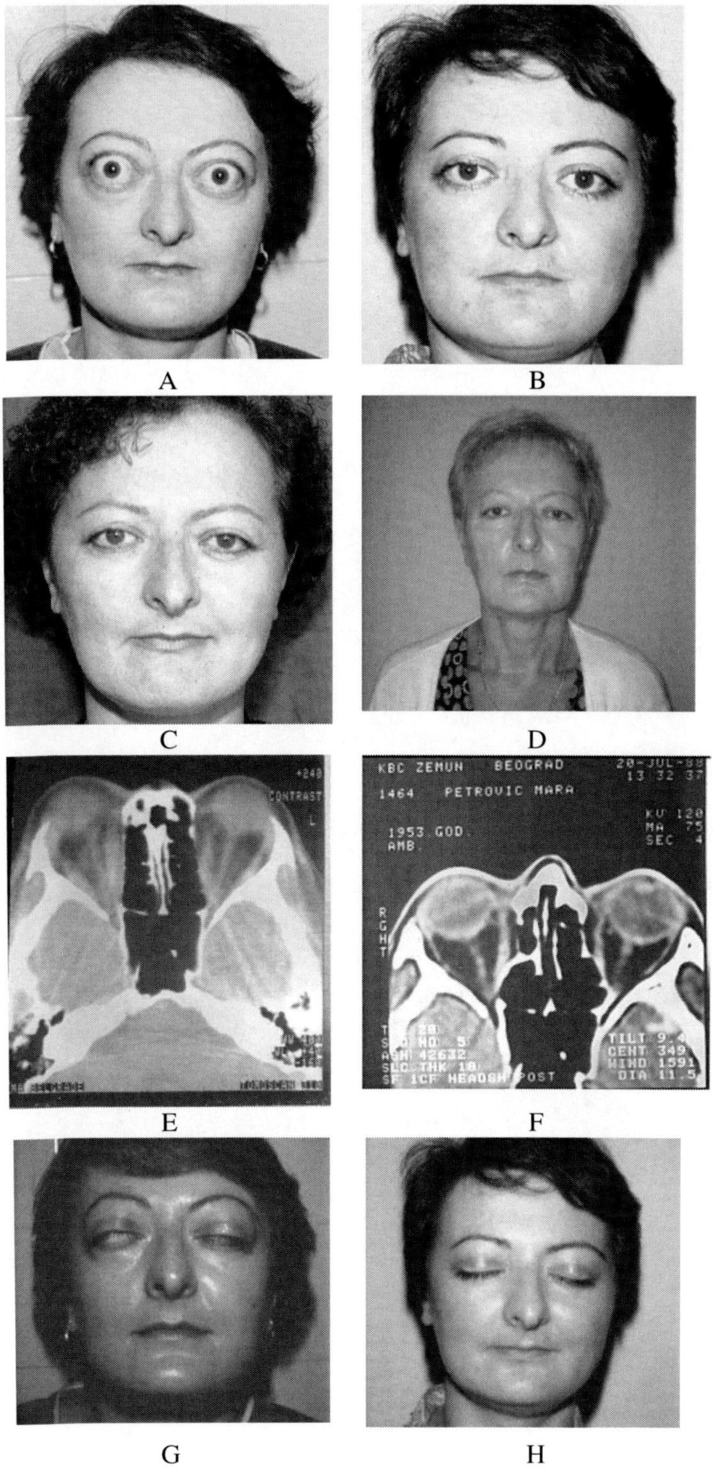

Figure 14. A. Patient with exophthalmos of 30 mm and eyelid retraction. B- One year after the operation. C. 9 years after the operation. D. 23 years atfer the operation. E, F. CT before and after the operation.G, H- Eye closing before and after the operation.

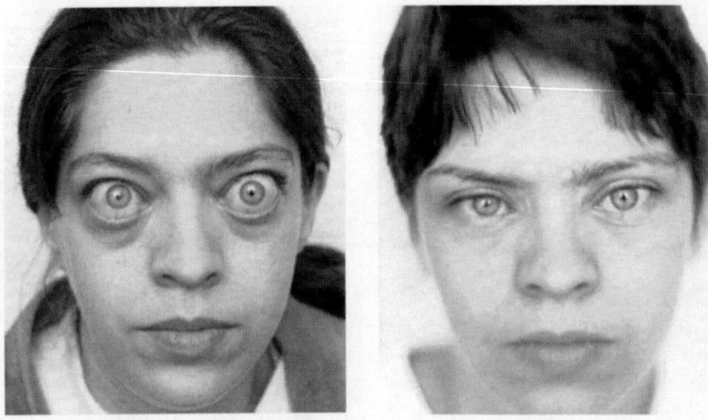

A B

Figure 15. A. Patient after thyroidectomy with exophthalmos of 32 mm, eyelid retraction and eyelid deformities (changes on the eyes are worsened after thyrodectomy). B. 3 months after the operation.

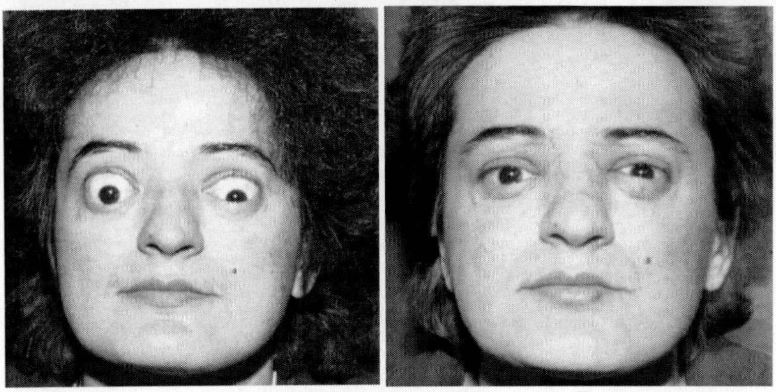

A B

Figure 16. A. Patient after inadequately antral-ethmoidal decompression with injury of extraocular muscles. B. 3 weeks after described decompression of the orbits and reconstruction of the anterior, bulbar part of orbital floors. It is necessary to perform additional correction of the left lower eyelid.

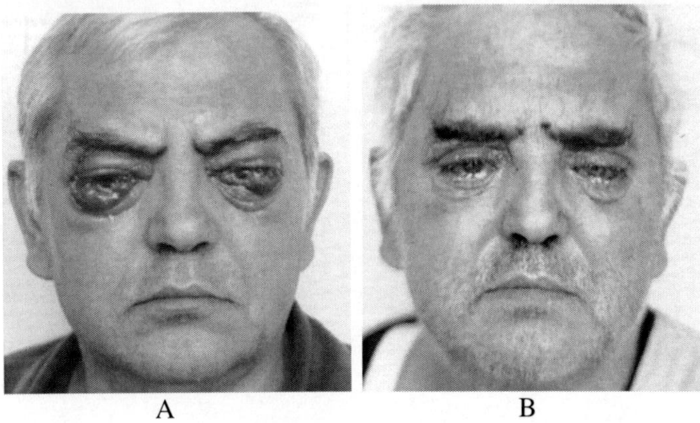

A B

Figure 17. A-Malignant DO with bilateral blindness. B. 7 days after the operation. The vision is improved significantly because of the recovery of the reversible changes of optic nerve and cornea.

4.4. Symptoms of Dysthyroid Ophthalmopathy

Due to previously specified changes on the organ of vision, dysthyroid ophthalmopathy has been followed by numerous symptoms. The most frequent difficulties start as eye scratch, which is manifested as "an eye full of sand." The scratching sensation is followed by photophobia and epiphora. These difficulties occur due to the damage on the epithelium of the cornea and the conjunctiva. Brief blurriness is the result of excessive tearing in the corneal area. The blurry morning vision is the result of disbalance in the extraocular muscles function. Permanent blurry vision, with defects in the visual field, is the consequence of the optic nerve damage. Double vision is the result of weakened function of the extraocular muscles due to their infiltration and thickening. At first, this occurs occasionally. Double vision usually appears in the morning and with a longer eye strain. With the advancement of the illness, fibrosis of the extraocular muscles causes the eye stiffness, strabismus and constant double vision. Almost all patients with dysthyroid ophthalmopathy complain of, a mild or a more severe, pressure-like pain deep down in the eyes. This pain can be explained by a rise in the intraorbital pressure and the pressure on the optic nerve. Many patients also complain of a more or less distinct dull pain in the forehead area. Dysthyroid ophthalmopathy can be accompanied by a high intraocular pressure – exogenous glaucoma (pseudoglaucoma), which is explained by an increased pressure of an enlarged orbital tissue on the eyeball.

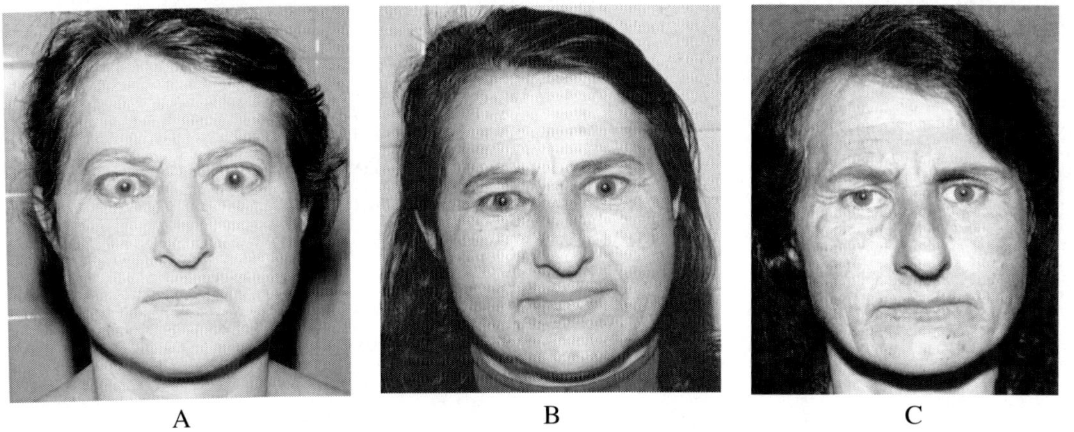

A B C

Figure 18. A. Patient with severe DO with steroid face, because of steroid therapy. B. 3 weeks after the operation. C. 6 years after the operation (without steroid therapy).

4.5. Diagnosistics of Dysthyroid Ophthalmopathy

In cases of a typical bilateral disease it is easy to give a diagnosis and it can be made "at the door." A unilateral exophthalmos in euthyroid persons represents somewhat a diagnositical problem and other diseases and changes in the orbit (tumors, vascular anomalies, orbital encephalocele, orbital inflammatory pseudotumors etc.) must be excluded. Although diagnosis in most cases is reached promptly, in order to obtain a true insight into the severity of the disease, numerous diagnostical methods must be applied. Inspection and palpation provide us with basic impressions. Biomicroscopy reveals changes on the conjunctiva and the cornea. Ophthalmoscopy reveals changes on the eye fundus. Tonometry determines the intraocular pressure. The visual acuity is determined by optotype cards. The degree of exophthalmos is determined by Hertel exophthalmometry. The disfunction of the extraocular muscles, accompanied by diplopia shall be determined by Hess-Lancaster test as a reliable method. The changes on the extraocular muscles, their thickening, changes on the orbital fat tissue, changes on the lacrimal gland, as well as the thickening of the periorbit and the optic nerve can be determined with great precision by echography. Computed tomography (CT) can determine with great precision the thickening of the muscles and the degree of exophthalmos on both sides, i.e., the length of the retrobulbar cone. Nuclear magnetic resonance (NMR) provides even more accurate data, fresh infiltrations of the extraocular muscles can be differentiated from fibrosis and degenerative changes.

4.6. Therapy of the Dysthyroid Ophthalmopathy

The treatment of hyperthyroidism often results in the improvement of the organ of vision. However, in many cases, although the stabilization of the thyroid gland function occurred and the patients were brought to euthyroid condition, the changes on the eyes would persist or even deteriorate. As it is known that dysthyroid ophthalmopathy occurs in a significant percentage of euthyroid persons, sometimes even hypothyroid, it should be clear that the therapy of this disease is uncertain and problematic.

The purpose of the conservative therapy – medicamentous and radiological – is to reduce the orbital and the periorbital swelling, thus causing a drop in the intraocular pressure. Medications used in this therapy are corticosteroids and immunosuppressants, with local instillation of various preparations. The combination of corticosteroids and immunosuppresants gives somewhat better results than each alone. The irradiation therapy is administered in patients not responding to the medications. There is also a possibility of combining medications and irradiation therapy.

The conservative therapy usually gives modest results and may cause various complications. Corticosteroids and immunosuppressants, if used in larger doses, may cause well-known general complications, whereas irradiation therapy may result in various local complications (keratopathy, iritis, cataract, retinopathy, optic neuropathy).

4.6.1. Surgical Therapy

Since conservative therapy of marked dysthyroid ophthalmopathy often does not give satisfactory results, surgical treatment is used more and more often nowadays. Surgical procedures include operations on the eyelids, operation on the extraocular muscles and different methods of orbital decompression. Tarsorrhaphy, i.e., blepharorrhaphy, partial or complete, is performed for the protection of the cornea, i.e., for the prevention of ulceration and perforation of the cornea. The upper eyelid retraction, that follows dysthyroid ophthalmopathy, can be surgically resolved by the excision of central part of the aponeurosis of the eyelid levator muscle and Müller's muscle [26-30]. With this procedure the exophthalmos is partially masked, the cornea is protected, and cosmetic effect is also achieved. For correction of the upper eyelid retraction, the method of graft interposition is often used. Operations on the lower eyelid muscle are rarely performed. When the lower eyelid is stretched and sagging because of a marked exophthalmos, it is possible to shorten the eyelid horizontally and lift it by performing the excision of the central part of the eyelid rim about 3 mm wide [26-30]. A better result can be achieved if the inferior tarsal stripe is fixed to the lateral orbital margin, i.e., if lateral cantopexy is performed [26-30]. In this manner, the lower eyelid is also lifted. The exophthalmos is slightly masked by this and cosmetic effect is achieved.

Operations on the extrabulbar muscles are performed with the purpose of correcting strabismus and double vision. Attitudes about the possibilities and indications for this surgical procedure are set out in the following pages.

4.6.1.1. Orbital Decompression

Orbital decompression is the most efficient method of dysthyroid ophthalmopathy treatment [2, 4, 8, 19, 21, 22, 25, 26-30, 34, 42]. Indications for orbital decompression are compressive optic neuropathy and marked exophthalmos followed by diplopia, keratopathy, ocular pressure, orbital pain, headache, epiphora and unattractive appearance of the patient. In most cases, a marked exophthalmos is accompanied by majority of the mentioned symptoms, However, even such a singular symptom, together with exophthalmos, may represent a major problem for most of patients, so if conservative therapy does not provide satisfactory results, orbital decompression is indicated. The degree of exophthalmos does not always correlate with the intensity of the symptoms and severity of disease. Often, in patients with distinct symptoms, even with a minor exophthalmos, orbital decompression is indicated as well. It is a big mistake to insist on the conservative therapy which does not give satisfactory results. Irreversible changes on the optic nerve and the extrabulbar muscles, i.e., papillary atrophy and fibrosis of the extrabulbar muscles should be avoided. In case of papillary atrophy, the improvement of vision can not be achieved by orbital decompression. If muscular fibrosis has been developed, it will be impossible to successfully correct strabismus and double vision by orbital decompression.

A number of orbital decompression methods have been applied so far, with more or less success. Dollinger [9] 1891 performed the first recorded orbital decompression by removing a portion of the lateral orbital wall. Hirsh and Urbaneck [13] 1930 proposed the removal of the orbital floor via transantral approach. Naffziger [23] 1931 introduced the concept of resection of the orbital roof via neurosurgical approach. Sewell [32] 1936 reported the resection of the medial orbital wall. Walsh and Ogura [38] 1957 introduced antral-ethmoidal decompression, i.e., removal of the orbital floor and medial wall via transantral approach. Tessier [34] 1969 and Wolfe [42] 1979 introduced the concept of orbital expansion, i.e., osteotomy of the anterior part of the orbital floor and lateral wall, after which that segment of the bone is moved frontward and fixed with wire ligatures in that position. In addition to the expansion, i.e., osteotomy and outward movement of the part of the lateral and the inferior orbital wall, Pearl and associates [25] also performed decompression on the medial orbital wall. Anderson and Lindberg 1981 [2] removed the orbital floor and medial wall via a translid approach. "Three-wall decompression" in which lateral wall decompression is added to antral-ethmoidal decompression and "four-wall decompression," described by Kennerdell and Maroon [17], in which removal of the lateral half of the orbital roof is added to "three-wall decompression" produce a better effect of decompression in comparison with previous methods. Bartalena et al. [4] 1989 remove the orbital roof, lateral wall and lateral part of the orbital floor using neurosurgical approach. Roncevic and Jackson [28] 1989 described a modified bilateral three-wall decompression via eyelids approach with removal of periorbital, intraorbital and retrobulbar fat along with the correction of the eyelid retraction and deformities. Olivari [24] 1991 reported unilateral, transpalpebral decompression by removal of the intraorbital fat. Krastinova et al. [19] 2006 remove the lateral and medial orbital walls using the coronal approach and lateral part of the orbital floor via lower eyelid. Nowadays, frequently endoscopic transnasal or transantral orbital decompression is applied.

In 2008. and 2010. author of this book gave a detailed description of the results achieved by his method of decompression on three walls, with the removal of the orbital fat tissue, with a simultaneous correction of the changes on the eyelids [26, 27]. Since this method constantly gives good functional and aesthetic results, it shall be described in detail below.

Decompression of the orbit is performed after a complete endocrine and ophthalmic assessment and treatment. The procedure for the correction begins within the upper eyelid (Figure 1). As for a blepharoplasty, the excision of the excessive eyelid skin and swollen subcutaneous tissue is performed and the eyelid fat and the fat from the upper part of the orbit is removed. In order to obtain the correction of the upper eyelid retraction, the central part of the aponeurosis of the levator muscle and Muller's muscle are excised. Following this, an incision is made in the lower eyelid, 2-3 mm below the margin. Through this subciliar incision, the floor and the lateral wall of the orbit are explored and the periorbital and intraorbital fat is removed, as much as possible. Using a small chisel and hemostat, the posterior, retrobulbar part of the orbital floor and the lateral orbital wall, with the exception of the lateral orbital margin, are removed (Figure 1). The bony bridge between the floor and the lateral wall defect is removed to produce a large continuous orbitectomy. The size of the defect is related to the severity of the ophthalmopathy and exophthalmos. An attempt should be made to remove the bone from the orbital floor as close to the orbital apex as possible. The anterior, bulbar part of the orbital floor should remain intact. The infraorbital nerve is protected during the floor osteotomy. This is achieved by removing the bone on either side and freeing the nerve afterwards. If the bone bridge in the infraorbital nerve region is left, the effect of decompression is significantly diminished. If possible, the sinus mucosa should not be opened. Small perforations of the sinus mucosa are frequently unavoidable, but are of no importance. Wide incisions or excisions of the periorbital periosteum should be made in several sites. Following this, through an incision made over the medial margin of the orbit, the medial orbital wall is explored and its ethmoidal part is removed (Figure 1). This medial wall bone defect should be in continuity with the orbital floor defect, i.e., retobulbar part of the orbital strut should be removed. During the medial orbital wall decompression, the bone at the region of the upper border of the ethmoid bone must be intact. The bone defect begins about 3 mm below the ethmoidal foramena. This is done in order to prevent injury and bleeding of the ethmoidal arteries and to prevent the breaking into scull cavity and damaging the dura. Using this same approach, the retrobulbar space is explored, and again, as much as possible, retrobulbar fat is removed with a hemostat. The periorbital periosteum in this region should be excised or incised at several sites. In patients with distended, hypotonic, ptotic lower eyelids it is necessary to perform the lateral canthopexy in order to correct these deformities. In some patients it is necessary to perform shortening of the lower eyelid by excision of the central part of the eyelid rim, about 3 mm wide. After establishment of satisfactory hemostasis, a thin vacuum drain is inserted into the retrobulbar space, and the skin incisions are closed. At the beginning of the operation, temporary blepharorrhaphy should be performed using two single sutures. These sutures are removed 5-7 days after the operation. Postoperatively the eyesight is controlled through central part of the eyelids, between the two sutures.

Significant symmetrical decompression, particularly in the narrow orbital apex, where there is the highest pressure, is achieved by the surgical treatment described. The elimination of this pressure is necessary for normalization of the function of all orbital structures, especially of the function of the optic nerve and extraocular muscles. In addition, if the retraction and eyelid swelling are corrected, all signs and symptoms of dysthyroid ophthalmopathy (DO) will disappear or will be significantly decreased. If it is performed with precision, this procedure is without high risk.

Of course, the main effect of decompression is achieved by the widening of the orbit, i.e., by the removal of the part of the orbital walls, especially in narrow apical region. Removal of the orbital fat has an additional effect, especially in cases with severe DO. The removal of fat only, without the removal of the part of the orbital walls [24], cannot produce satisfactory decompression in cases with marked DO [3, 26-30]. In certain patients with more evident exophthalmos, the orbital fat is atrophic, degenerated, so the removal of this small amount of the fat does not give a significant decompression and result. In some patients with asymmetric exophthalmos there is a smaller amount of fat on the side with more evident exophthalmos than on the other side. So, the main cause of exophthalmos are swollen, elongated extraocular muscles [26-30]. If the volume of orbital fat would be determinant of the eye position, numerous patients with severe DO would have enophthalmos due to atrophy of orbital fat. The statement, often emphasized, that the removal of 1cc of orbital fat means the reduction of exophthalmos by 1 mm, is not correct. Regadless, it is necessary to remove orbital fat, i.e., sick tissue, as much as possible. If DO is an autoimmune process, it is possible that important, if not main, autoimmune process occurs in the orbital fat.

Four-wall decompression [16] can provide some disadvantages. The surgical procedure lasts longer, a part of the brain can prolapse through the opening in the orbital roof which leads do a decrease in the orbital volume, causing a pulsatile eye or pulsatile exophthalmos (Figure 11). Transcranial, transfrontal approach [4] with the removal of the roof, the lateral wall and lateral part of the orbital floor can produce the same complications. Besides, this approach has a poorer decompression effect compared with four- wall decompression. Tough, it is difficult to believe that the four-wall decompression has a significantly greater decompression effect in comparison with the three-wall decompression, considering that dura, i.e., the brain, lies against the opening in the orbital roof. Also, it is difficult to believe that this method can produce the globe retrodisplacement from 14 to 16 mm [17, 22] i.e., 10 to 17 mm [33]. Globe retrodisplacement depends not only on the bony opening, i.e., increased orbital volume, but also on the amount of periostal openings and the condition of orbital tissues, especially on the condition of extraocular muscles.

In order to obtain the functional, as well as the aesthetic effect of decompression, even in severe cases of DO, it is enough to achieve globe retrodisplacemnet ranging from 7 to 9 mm which can be done using the method described. Globe retodisplacement ranging from 14 to 16 or 17 mm almost always leads to marked enophthalmos and malposition of the eyes with strabismus and diplopia.

Antal-ethmoidal decompression [36, 38] and all other previously used methods [9, 13, 23, 32] are archaic methods, providing inadequate results and poor visibility during operation.

In the majority of up-to-now applied methods of orbital decompression, the orbital floor is frequently removed in conjunction with medial or lateral wall decompression. Leone et al. [21] recommended medial and lateral wall decompression with the removal of the lateral orbital rim. They claim that the removal of the orbital floor causes postoperative complications "involving extraocular muscle imbalance, infraorbital anaesthesia, hypo-ophthalmia, and recurrent sinusitis." Decompression of the lateral wall of the orbit produces a relatively small effect. Removal of the lateral rim does not lead to decompression of extraocular muscles and optic nerve, but there is always a visible deformity. If only posterior, retrobulbar part of orbital floor is removed, it is practically impossible to produce hypo-ophthalmia. If orbital decompression is performed with precision, residual diplopia is the consequence of the initial disease process and not of the operation. The same will occur by decompression of only the medial and lateral walls if the preoperative exophthalmos was marked with diplopia. In such cases, there will be more frequent residual diplopia because of insufficient decompression. If the surgery is performed carefully it is quite possible to avoid serious injury to the infraorbital nerve. After decompression of the orbital floor, if the sinus mucosa is injured, the sinus will be filled with blood. Blood clots in the sinus are eliminated spontaneously through the natural sinus ostium as happens after facial bone injuries and orthognathic surgery. None of the patients from the group presented on the end of this chapter have had a sinusitis so far. Thus, there is no reason to avoid decompression of orbital floor, i.e., removal of the whole retrobulbar part. Without this procedure it is impossible to achieve adequate decompression of the orbital apex, and it is virtually impossible to get good functional and aesthetic results in cases of severe DO.

If only the lateral part of the orbital floor is removed using the Bartalena [4] and Krastinova [19] methods, it is equally impossible to achieve good orbital decompression since the medial part of the orbital floor (medially from infraorbital nerve) is considerably larger than the lateral part. In some cases, in order to perform orbital enlargement and better correction of exophthalmos, Krastinovaet al. [19] insert the calvarial bone transplants on the lateral and superior orbital rim and the nasal bone. The mentioned enlargement makes AP diameter of the orbit longer. Longer diameter of the orbit effects stronger pressure in the apical region of the orbit, which is certainly unfavourable for further course of the disease.

It is true that by applying the method described by Pearl et al. [25] the orbit is widened in its anterior part and its volume is increased, but this procedure gives a poor decompression effect on the orbital apex where the main problem lies. Similarly, orbital expansion by Tessier [34] and Wolfe [42], along with the visible face deformity, does not give satisfactory decompression in the orbital apex.

The endoscopic transnasal or transantral orbital decompresion is less traumatic procedure than classic surgical methods of the orbital decompression. But, with this technique it is impossible to perform wide three wall decompression and the removal of significant amount of orbital fat, i.e., it is essentially impossible to achieve good result in the cases of the marked DO. After the endoscopic decompression of the orbit the patients often have worsening of diplopa. The transconjunctival decompression has the disadvantages similar to endoscopic decompression.

In cases of emergency Krastinova et al. [19] emphasize: "expansion must be minimally invasive to save vision without risking an overcorrection of the proptosis in cases of a secondary regression of the ophthalmopathy." In emergency cases (Figures 13, 17) we deal with severe cases of DO and it is necessary to perform wide three wall decompression with preservation of anterior, bulbar part of the orbital floor. If the expansion is performed correctly, overcorrection of the proptosis is virtually impossible. In response to the letter regarding this paper Krastinova et al. emphasize that in emergency cases, through a subtarsal, "minimally invasive" or "direct approach," they remove "entire orbital floor" and emphasize: "Even in these cases, we try to spare the infraorbital nerve." Removal of the entire orbital floor during this "minimally invasive" expansion inevitably leads to the overcorrection, enophthalmos, malposition of the eyes with strabismus and diplopia. The infraorbital nerve can be and must always be preserved.

It has been frequently stated that orbital decompression does not usually improve extraocular muscle function and that after the operation, there is often a deterioration of extraocular muscle function. Waller et al. [37] claim that decompression does not, as a rule, improve muscle function, that muscle dysfunction and diplopia were more apparent after the operation in the majority of cases, and that nearly 70% of their total group of patients required one or more strabismus operations after orbital decompression. Shorr et al. [33] state that they had 34% incidence of worsened muscle balance after orbital decompression. Similar statements have been made by De Santo [8]. Garrity et al. [10] emphasize that after transantral orbital decompression in 428 patients, "postoperatively new diplopia developed in 74 (64%) of 116 patients who had no diplopia before orbital decompression, although 300 patients ultimately had strabismus surgery." Adenis et al. [1] report that all patients with moderate or severe diplopia remained with diplopia after fat removal orbital decompression and that 32% operated patients developed a new diplopia. Russo et al. [31] state that, after 3-wall orbital decompression, in 18% of patients with diplopia there was no modification of diplopia and that in 23,5% of patients a more severe imbalance occurred. Kasperbauer and Hinkley [16] report that only 25% of their patients "did not require eye muscle surgery" after endoscopic decompression of the orbit.

What could be the cause of non-improvement and even deterioration of extraocular muscle function after orbital decompression? The main cause, beside fibrosis of the muscles, appears to be inadequate and insufficient orbital decompression. DO is complex pathological condition with serious pathological changes of all tissues of the orbital contents and the eyelids. Decompression of the orbit has numerous important details. Even one inadequately performed detail can be the cause for poor postoperative results, especially regarding diplopia and strabismus.

The majority of those who emphasize the poor function of the extraocular muscles after decompression of the orbit, performed this operation via transantral or endoscopic approach. By applying transantral approach, due to poor visibility in the course of the operation, it is possible to injure the extraocular muscles and cause a worsening of their function. If anterior, bulbar part of the orbital floor is removed, by any approach, the globe loses its support and drops toward the sinus (Figure 16), which results in worsening of the strabismus and diplopia. Moreover, if the operation is performed in such a way, the pressure in the orbital apex remains, and a sufficient decompression effect, which would enable improvement in extraocular muscle function, is not achieved. In general, if the pressure in the orbital apex is not eliminated, a considerable improvement in extraocular muscle function and optic nerve function cannot be expected. Also, removal of the orbital fat contributes to a decrease in pressure in the orbit and an improvement in the optic nerve function and extraocular muscle function. Though lateral decompression gives the least effect of decompression, it should also be performed in all the cases of decompression through the floor and medial wall. Lateral decompression, in addition prevents superfluous medial globe displacement which can also cause worsening of diplopia. The openings made in all orbital walls should be continuous, without bone bridges between the walls, as well as in the region of the infraorbital nerve. In this way an important symmetrical decompression is achieved which enables the recovery of the optic nerve and balanced decompression, i.e., the recovery of the extraocular muscle. Unbalanced recovery of the extraocular muscles can worsen diplopia.

Strabismus operations should not be performed before orbital decompression. If orbital decompression is not performed before the strabismus operation, the latter will only lead to temporary improvement in extraocular muscle function, because it does not solve basic condition for extraocular muscle recovery. Strabismus surgery should not be performed during the decompression of the orbit as well, because of a real possibility of spontaneous recovery of the extraocular muscles function after decompression (Figures 4, 7, 8, 10, 13, 16). If spontaneous recovery, supported by exercises of eye movements, does not occur three months after operation, a strabismus operation is indicated. The first day after orbital decompression, it is necessary to start with exercises of the eye movements to prevent fibrosis, scar around extraocular muscles, which can limit the function of the muscles and be the cause of diplopia.

The majority of authors who write about orbital decompression, perform the correction of the eyelid retraction in the second operation. For correction of the eyelid retraction, technique of graft interposition is mainly used. The authors do not discuss what has been done with regards to the correction of eyelid deformities, which have always been the part of DO. Using the described method of orbital decompression and correction of eyelid deformities, it is possible to perform decompression of the orbits and correction of eyelid retraction and deformities, with very good, even excellent results, in single operation, i.e., it is possible to avoid numerous operations. In cases when the lacrimal gland is swollen and enlarged, it is impossible to obtain good aesthetic results of eyelid correction if the part of the gland, which protrudes beyond the orbit, is not excised. After this procedure the patients do not have a significant diminution of the tear production. Of course, if patient has "dry eyes," which is rare, this procedure is not indicated.

The temporary blepharorrhaphy, which is performed at the beginning of the operation, protects the globe during the operation and during the first 5-7 days after the operation. Besides, blepharorrhaphy produces a slight pressure on the globe, which has an influence on moving the globe into the newly created space.

The blepharorrhaphy, which is used by some in shorter or longer intervals, in cases of severe DO, in order to protect cornea and to soothe swelling and infection of the conjunctiva, should be maximally avoided. Exophthalmos is a kind of spontaneous decompression. If blepharorrhaphy is performed, the pressure in the orbit, especially in the orbital apex increases and leads to a faster damaging of the optic nerve and extraocular muscles. It increases intraocular pressure and deteriorates some subjective problems such is headaches and the pain in the eyes and the orbits.

4.7. Complications of Decompression of the Orbit and Their Prevention

Orbital decompression is a serious and complex operation. In the course of orbital decompression various immediate postoperative complications may occur. Diplopia, and mistakes in the course of the operation causing aggravation of diplopia have already been discussed. In the course of correction of upper eyelid retraction, i.e., excision of central part of the levator muscle aponeurosis and Muller's muscle, if the excision is performed inadequately, eyelid ptosis can occur. During the decompression of the orbital floor, the infraorbital nerve may be damaged or cut. However, even when this nerve has not been damaged, in most of the operated patients hypoesthesia or anesthesia of the infraorbirtal region occurs postoperatively, lasting for several days, weeks or months. There are several reasons for this. The most important is the traumatization of the infraorbital nerve during the removal of the surrounding bone, and the pressure of the eye and orbital tissue on the nerve which remained bare after removal of the surrounding bone, i.e., out of its groove or sulcus. Should the decompression of the floor and medial wall in the apical part of the orbit not be done with a great precision, the optic nerve may be damaged or cut. The damage of the optic nerve and the central artery and vein of retina may also occur during a rough extirpation of the orbital fat, particularly the retrobulbar part of this tissue. Should the anterior, bulbar part of the orbital floor be removed, the eye shall drop towards maxillary sinus (Figure 16) with all the consequences resulting from such a position of the eye. During decompression of the medial orbital wall it is possible to cause injury of the anterior and posterior ethmoidal arteries if the procedure is performed above the frontoethmoidal suture. If these arteries become injured, cauterization must be performed by a bipolar cautery. Should the procedure be performed above the frontoethmoidal suture, it shall be possible to perforate the cribriform lamina and dura, with occurrence of CSF in the nose. The amount of the fluid depends on the degree of dura injury. It must be kept in mind that sometimes the cribriform lamina has been anatomically lowered towards the ethmoid sinus, so the injury of this lamina and dura may occur even when the trepanation of the ethmoid sinus, i.e., decompression on the orbital medial wall has been properly performed, i. e. below the frontoethmoidal suture. In order to avoid that, trepanation of the ethmoidal sinus must be performed 3 mm below the frontoethmoidal suture. In the course of decompression on the lateral orbital wall by removing a part of the zygomatic bone behind the lateral orbital margin, communication is established with the temporal and infratemporal region. A part of the Bishat's fat pad prolapses into the orbit through this communication. This part of the fat must be removed, so that the effect of decompression is not diminished. In the course of the operation, the lacrimal drainage apparatus may be injured or interrupted. In order to avoid this, the incision on the medial margin of the orbit should stretch from medial part of the eyebrow to the level of the medial corner of the eye. Should this incisions go lower, the lacrimal drainage apparatus may be injured, as well as medial ligament. In the early postoperative period a large blood clot can be formed in the retrobulbar space which, by its pressure on the optic nerve, may cause blindness. In order to avoid this, a vacuum drain should be inserted into the retrobulbar space. The drain should be left there 24 hours. In patients having pansinusitis or a chronic inflammation of the nasal mucosa, and in those who had injury of dura during decompression, with the occurrence of CSF, meningitis may develop in the postoperative period. In spite of the present chronic pansinusitis, in the patient in Figure 6, described orbital decompression is performed due to the changes on the eyes and the threat of blindness. For the last 22 years there have been no serious problems, specially concerning meningitis. In the early postoperative period the orbital infection may also be developed if during operation the aseptic and antiseptic measures have not been applied. For the purpose of preventing orbital infection, an adequate antibiotic therapy must be introduced. This therapy should be started immediately prior to the operation. In the course of the operation, the application of steroid therapy should be initiated, which shall be resumed postoperatively for 7-10 days with a gradual dose reduction. This therapy has an affect on diminishing the swelling of the eyelids and the orbital tissue, recovery of the extraocular muscles is boosted and a quick development of a fibrous tissue in the region of decompressing bone openings on the orbital walls is prevented. If soon after the operation connective tissue gets formed in the decompressing openings in the orbital walls, the result of the operation, i.e., decompression shall be considerably diminished. For faster recovery of the function of the extrabulbar muscle Dexason can be injected directly into the muscle during the operation.

The described method of orbital decompression by author of this book stems from an understanding of the pathology, is less hazardous, relatively easy to perform, gives constantly good functional and aesthetic results and allows rapid recovery.

4.8. Patients and Results of Surgical Therapy

Since year 1986, 119 patients with severe TO (exophthalmos 24-33 mm) were treated surgically, by the author, using described method of the orbital decompression along with correction of the eyelid retraction and deformities. There were 91 women of the ages 17 to 73 years and 28 men of ages 22 to 53. In all cases, except the 3 cases of unilateral disease, the operation was performed on both orbits in a single operation. After the operation, in different time intervals, subjective symptoms were observed in all the patients and the changes in the eyelids, conjunctiva and cornea recorded. Degree of exophthalmos by Hertel, the function of extraocular muscles, i.e., diplopia by Hess-Lancaster test, intraocular pressure, the change in the disc, changes in vision and field of vision, as well as the thickening and elongation of extraocular muscles by CT, MRI scan or echography were also monitored.

Using described method of orbital decompression, all symptoms and manifestations of DO disappeared or were significantly decreased. Although the results are evident immediately after the operation, definitive results were obtained in 2 to 3 months thereafter. Complete comparisons of the preoperative and postoperative results were conducted in 65 patients three months after the operation. Postoperatively, in all patients subjective symptoms were considerably reduced or have disappeared. The swelling and deformities of the eyelids disappeared or were significantly reduced. Due to unsatisfactory correction of the upper eyelid retraction it was necessary to perform lengthening of the upper eyelid in four patients and correction of lower eyelid deformity in three patients. Conjunctival hyperemia and chemosis, as well as exposure keratitis resolved in all patients. All patients showed a significant reduction of exophthalmos (5-11 mm, 7.2 mm on average) with marked improvement or normalization of ocular muscle function (Figures 2-18, Tables 3, 4). There were no cases of subsequent impairment of ocular motility, diplopia or strabismus. Due to unsatisfactory correction of double vision and because of residual diplopia, strabismus surgery was performed in six patients. Out of 129 DO orbits in which decompression was performed, there was impairment of vision in 67 eyes due to optic neuropathy and/or due to corneal change. After the operation, the majority of these patients (68%) showed improvement of vision and improvement or elimination of the field defect (Table 5). In all patients with partial atrophy of the disc and irreversible changes in the cornea, there was no improvement in vision. In only one patient the subsequent unilateral impairment of vision occurred. The intraocular pressure measured by mmHg before the operation was 12 to 30, mostly 23 to 27, the average being 23. After the operation the pressure was 12 to 23, mostly 12 to 19, average being 15. Until now, less evident relapse was recorded in only 3 cases out of total patients group and in only one patient unilateral reoperation was required (removal of fibrous tissue from the bony defects of the orbital walls, which were done in the previous surgery, as well as eventual widening of these bony defects). Echography, CT and MRI scans showed great reduction of extraocular muscle thickening and shortening of the retrobulbar cone in all operated patients. Finally, significant aesthetic improvement has been achieved in all patients (Figures 2-18). Having followed these patients for years, the mentioned results, sustained with adequate endocrinological therapy, were stable.

Table 3. Changes of exophthalmos 3 months after orbital decompression (n = 129)

Reduction in mm.	Number of eyes
5	11
6	24
7	48
8	29
9	11
10	4
11	2

Table 4. Diplopia before and 3 months after the orbital decompression (n = 65)

	Without diplopia	Diplpia upward or/and lateral gaze	Diplopia on straight gaze
Before operation	17	33	15
After operation	43	16	6

Table 5. Vision changes 3 months after orbital decompression (n = 67)

Improvement	46
Unchanged	21
Impairment	0/1

Complications: The majority of patients had transient hypoesthesia or anesthesia of the infraorbital region. In one patient there was unilateral loss of vision a week after the operation. The ophthalmological consult conclusion was that the reason for the loss of vision was the embolism of the central artery of retina. One patient with chronic rhinitis had meningitis, with improvement after antibiotic therapy. One patient had nasal CSF with spontaneous disappearance during one week.

Conclusion

Conservative therapy in cases of severe forms of disthyroid ophthalmopathy does not give satisfactory results. In such cases orbital decompression is indicated in order to prevent irreversible changes of the optic nerve, cornea and the extraocular muscles, and also to eliminate or reduce subjective ailments. Decompression of the floor, the medial and the lateral orbital wall, with the removal of the periorbital, intraorbital and retrobulbar fat tissue results in a significant drop of pressure in the orbit, particularly in the apex, which enables decongestion, i.e., recovery of the bulbomotor muscle and the optic nerve, and a significant reduction of the exophthalmos. During the same surgical procedure it is possible to successfully remove the swollen eyelid tissue and correct the eyelid retraction. If this operation is performed with precision, permanently good results can be expected, both functional and aesthetic, and the risk of serious complications is relatively small.

References

[1] Adenis, JP; Camezind, P; Robert, PY., Is incidence of diplopia after fat removal orbital Decompression predictive factor of choice of surgical technique for Graves ophthalmopathy. *Bull.Acad.Natl.Med.* 2003, 187:1649-1658,2003.

[2] Anderson R. L., Linberg J. V., Transantral approach to decompression in Graves' disease, *Arch. Ophthalmol.* 99: 120-124, 1981.

[3] Baldeshi L., Boshi A., Orbital decompression in thyroid eye disease. In: Medel L., Vasquez L. M., editors, Orbital surgery, Basel, Karger, 2014, pp 18-33.

[4] Bartalena L., Marcocci., Bogazzi F., Panicuccu M., Bruno-Bossio G., Orbital decompression for severe Graves' ophthalmopathy. *J. Neurosurg. Sci.* 33: 223–227, 1989.

[5] Braverman L. E., Prevention of thyroid eye disease and final conclusion. *Thyroid* 8: 453 – 454, 1998.

[6] Chair D. H., Thyroid eye disease. Wiliam and Wilkins, Baltimore, 1985.

[7] Chen B, Shanli T, Smith TJ. IL-1 induces IL-6 expression in human orbital fibroblast: Identification of an anatomic-site specific phenotypic attribute relevant to thyroid-associated ophthalmopathy. *J Immunol* 175:1310-1319., 2005.

[8] De Santo L. W., The total rehabilitation of Graves' disease. *Laryngoscope* 90: 1652 - 1678, 1980.

[9] Dollinger J., Die Druckentlastung der Augenhohle durch Entfernung der ausseren Orbitawand bei hochgradigem Exophtalamus (Morbus Besedowi) und konsekutiver Hornhauterkrankung. Dtsch. Med. Wochenschr. 37: 1888 – 1890, 1911.

[10] Garrity, JA; Fatourechi, V; Bergstralh, EJ; Bartley, GB; Beathy, CW; DeSanto, LW; Gorman, CA. Results of transantral orbital decompression in 428 patients with severe Graves' orbitopathy. *Am. J. Ophthalmol.* 116: 533-547. 1993.

[11] Graves R.J., Enlargement of thyroid gland. Clinical lectures. *Med.Surg. J.*7:516–523, 1835.

[12] Heufelder AF. Pathogenesis of Graves'ophthalmopathy: Recent controversies and prognosis. *Eur J Endocrinol* 132:532-541, 1995.

[13] Hirsh V.O., Urbaneck J., Behanbdlung eines exzessiven Exophthalmus (Basedow) durch Entfernung von Orbitalfett von der Kieferhole aus, Monatsschr. *Ohrheilkd. Laryngorhinol.* 64: 212 – 213, 1930.

[14] Kanski J.J., The eye in systematic disease, Butterworths, London, 1986, p. 1 -9.

[15] Karageorgos g., Papadam A.J., Kollia G., Karalis D., Thyroid ophthalmopathy: 20 years experience with the treatment, *Thyroid* 8: 461 – 462, 1998.

[16] Kasperbauer, JL; Hinkley, L. Endoscopic orbital decompression for Graves ophthalmopathy. *Am. J. Rhinology*, 2005, 19, 603-605.

[17] Kennerdell J. S., Maroon J.C., An orbital decopression for severe dysthyroid exophthalmos, *Ophthalmology* 89: 467 – 472, 1982.

[18] Komarowsky J, Stepien H. Imuno-pathogenesis of thyroid associated ophthalmopathy [TAO]: The effect of novel treatment of TAO with TNFa and anti-CD monoclonal antibodies. In: Mertens L, Bogaert J, editors, Handbook of Hyperthyroidism, etiology, diagnosis, treatment. New York: Nova Science Publisher; 2010. pp 345-357.

[19] Krastinova-Lolov D, Bach CA, Hartl DM. Surgical strategy in the treatment of globe protrusion depending on its mechanism (Graves'Disease, nonsyndromic exorbitism, or high myopia). *Plast Reconstr Surg* 117:553-564, 2006.

[20] Lazarus J. H., Relation between thyroid eye disease and type of treatment of Graves' hyperthyroidism, *Thyroid* 8: 437 – 438, 1998.

[21] Leone C.R. Jr., Piest K. L., Newman R. J., Medial and lateral wall decompression for thyroid ophthalmopathy, *Am. J. Opthalmol.* 108: 160 – 166, 1989.

[22] McCord C. D. Jr., Current trends in orbital decompression, *Ophthalmology* 92: 21 – 23, 1985.

[23] Naffziger H. C., Progressive exophthalamus following thyroidectomy: its pathology and treatment *Ann. Surg.* 94: 582 – 568, 1931.

[24] Olivari N., Transpalpebral decompression of endocrine ophthalmopathy (Graves disease) by removal of intraorbital fat, *Plast. Reconstr. Surg.* 87: 621- 641, 1991.

[25] Pearl R. M., Vistenes l., Troxel S., Treatment of exophthalmos, Plast. Reconst. Surg. 87: 236 – 244, 1991.

[26] Roncevic R., Correction of exophthalmos and eyelid deformities in patients with severe thyroid ophthalmopathy, experience for 20 years. *J. Craniofacial Surg.* 19:628-636,2008.

[27] Roncevic R., Results of orbital decompression in patients with severe thyroid ophthalmopaty – experience of 22 years. In: Mertens J., Bogaert J. editors, Handbook of Hiperthyroidism, etiology, diagnosis, treatment, New York, Nova Science Publisher, 2010, pp. 129-158.

[28] Rončević R., Jackson I. T., Surgical treatment of thyrotoxic exophthalmos, *Plast. Reconstr. Surg*. 84: 754 – 760, 1989.

[29] Rončević R., Rončević D., Surgical treatment of severe dysthyroid ophthalmopathy – long term results, *J. Craniomaxillofac. Surg*. 23: 355 – 362, 1995.

[30] Roncevic R., Savkovic Z., Roncevic D., Results of diplopia and strabismus in patients with severe thyroid ophthalmopathy after orbital decompression, *Indian J. Ophthalmol.* 62:266-273,2014.

[31] Russo, V; Querques, G; Primavera, V; Della Noci, N. Incidence and treatment of diplopia after three –wall orbital decompression in Graves' ophthalmopathy. *J. Pediatr. Ophthalmol. Strabismus*, 41:219-225,2004.

[32] Sewell E. C., Operative control of progressive exophthalmos, *Arch. Otolaryngol*. 24: 621 – 624, 1936.

[33] Shorr N., Neuhaus R. W., Baylis H. I., Ocular motility problems after orbital decompression for dysthyroid ophthalmopathy, *Ophthalmology* 89: 323 – 328, 1982.

[34] Tessier P., Les exophthalmies. Expansion chirurgicale de l'orbite, *Ann. Chir. Plast*. 14: 207 – 214, 1969.

[35] Trobe J.D., Glaser J.S., LaFlamme P., Dysthyroid optic neuropathy, *Arch. Ophthalmopathy* 96: 1199 – 1209.

[36] Thawley S. E., Ogura J., Jacobs J., Transantral approach for orbital decompression, in Smith B.C., Ophthalmic Plastic and Reconstructive Surgery, Mosby, St. Louis, 1987, p. 1393 -1400.

[37] Waller R.R., de Santo L. W., Anderson R.I., Management of thyroid ophthalmopathy, in: Smith B.C., Ophthalmic Plastic and Reconstructive Surgery, Mosby, St. Louis, 1987, p. 1369 -2392.

[38] Walsh T. E., Ogura J. H., Transantral orbital decompression for malignant exophthalmos, *Laryngoscope* 64: 544 -568, 1957.

[39] Werner S. C., Modification of the classification of the eye changes of Graves' disease, *Am. J. Ophthalmol*. 83: 725 – 727, 1977.

[40] Wiersinga W. M., Graves' ophthalmopathy, in: Henneman G., Krenning E.P., Thyroid International, pamphlet No. 3, p. 3-15, Merck KgaA, Darmstadt, 1997.

[41] Wiersinga MW, Prummel MF. Pathogenesis of Graves' ophthalmopathy - current understanding. *J Clin Endocrinol Metab* 86:501-504, 2001.

[42] Wolfe S.A., Modified three-wall orbital expansion to correct persistent exophthalmos or exorbitism, *Plast. Reconstr. Surg*. 64: 448 -455, 1979.

[43] Young L. S., Henkind P., Medical aspects of Graves' ophthalmopathy, in: Smith B.C., Ophthalmic Plastic and Reconstructive Surgery, Mosby, St. Louis, 1987, p.1362.

Chapter 5

Lacrimal Apparatus Surgery

5.1. Introduction

The lacrimal apparatus consists of the lacrimal gland, the minor lacrimal glands, the lacrimal canaliculi, the lacrimal sac and the nasolacrimal duct. Any serious change, i.e., anomaly on any part of the lacrimal system, congenital or acquired, shall cause a major or minor dysfunction of this system [1-8].

The most frequent congenital anomalies are aplasia or hypoplasia of certain parts of the lacrimal apparatus, as well as obstructions of the lacrimal points, the lacrimal canaliculi or the nasolacrimal duct. The acquired anomalies of the lacrimal system are the consequence of injuries, inflammations, tumors and of various operations on parts of the lacrimal system or on the surrounding regions.

Many of the lacrimal apparatus anomalies mentioned here can be surgically corrected with restoring a partial or total functionality of the lacrimal system.

5.2. Diagnosis of Lacrimal Apparatus Disorders

The diagnosis of various disorders in the lacrimal system function is obtained on the basis of clinical history, inspection and palpation of the orbit, the eyelids and the nasal cavity, by probing and irrigation of the lacrimal system, X-ray, ultrasound, CT, MRI images, as well as scintigraphy and biopsy.

Clinical history provides information about the patient's ailments, particularly about the lacrimation disorders i.e., whether the patient lacrimates constantly, occassionally, during exertion or when crying.

Based on inspection it shall be determined whether the eyes are dry, whether the patient lacrimates and whether there are visible anomalies in the lacrimal system, such as the insufficient number of lacrimal points etc. By the inspection of the nasal cavum different pathological conditions can be seen (tumors, inflammations, deviation of the nasal septum etc.) which cause the obstruction of the nasolacrimal excretory ducts.

Tumors can be felt by palpation. If mucoid or mucopurulent content drains at the lacrimal points during the pressure on the lacrimal sac, most likely there is obstruction of the nasolacrimal duct. Because of the obstruction the lacrimal sac can be more or less dilated, and sometimes even inflamed with the inflammation of the facial soft tissues surrounding the sac.

Probing and irrigation of the lacrimal system give the information about obstruction of the lacrimal points, the lacrimal canaliculi, the lacrimal sac and the nasolacrimal duct. If the liquid has been discharged into the nose by irrigation, without a reflux, the lacrimal system is passable. Total reflux indicates a total obstruction, while a partial reflux, with partial passing of the liquid into the nose indicates a major or minor stricture in the lacrimal system.

Ultrasound, X-ray, CT, MRI diagnostics, as well as scintigraphy indicate the position, size and often the nature of the pathological process (tumors, inflammations, stones, anatomic anomalies etc.). Dacryocystography with contrast provides information about the lumen of the lacrimal canaliculi, the lacrimal sac and the nasolacrimal duct, and about the place of obstruction or stricture.

Biopsy of certain pathological processes provides information about their nature.

5.3. Surgical Therapy

5.3.1. Lacrimal Gland Surgery

Most often the reasons for surgical intervention on the lacrimal gland are various benign and malignant tumors. The approach to the lacrimal gland is achieved by the anterior orbitotomy through the incision on the eyelid or through the eyebrow, or by the lateral orbitotomy. These approaches are described in the chapter "Surgery of the Orbital Tumors." If the malignant tumor of the lacrimal gland has been infiltrated into the orbit, then most often the exenteration of the orbit has been indicated. In more severe cases of dysthyroid ophthalmopathy the lacrimal gland has been significantly swollen and enlarged and protrudes outside the orbit. For the purpose of good aesthetics of the eyelid correction, the part of the gland protruding outside the orbit should be excised [7]. Such excision of the part of the gland shall not cause disorder in the secretion and drainage of tears.

5.3.2. Lacrimal Canaliculi Surgery

Congenital absence of the lacrimal canaliculi or rudimentary canaliculi, strictures or obstructions of the canaliculi, and various traumatic injuries require a surgical therapy. The strictures of the canaliculi occur as a result of a chronical infection, antiglaucomatous, polychemo and irradiation therapy or trauma. If the canaliculi are intubated by the Jones' silicon tube in the early phase, i.e., in the beginning of the formation of a stricture, their function can be preserved [4, 5, 6]. When the strictures are well developed and diffused, in cases of canaliculi obstruction, as well as in the cases of congenital aplasia of the canaliculi and the lacrimal points, conjunctivodacryocystorhinostomy must be performed [2, 4, 5, 6]. Traumatic cutting of the canaliculi requires intubation of the Jones' sillicone tube, through which the parts of the canaliculi are attached together and stitched by a Vicryl or similar suture of 7-0 or 8-0 [1, 2, 4, 5, 6] (Figure 1). In case of obstruction, the narrow part of the canaliculi, the place of obstruction is excised, a sillicone tube is placed into the canaliculi through which the parts of the canaliculi are connected and stitched as described. Probing, i.e bougienage of the canaliculi rarely gives good results. After this procedure, the Jones' silicone tube should be placed into the canaliculi.

5.3.3. Surgery of Lacrimal SAC and Nasolacrimal Duct

Acute inflamations of the lacrimal sac are most often treated by incision and antibiotics. In case of chronic inflamation such therapeutic procedure, generally, has no effect and therefore dacryocystorhinostomy is required. In cases of tumor, the extirpation of the lacrimal sac is indicated. The extirpation of the affected lacrimal sac is also indicated in cases of ozaena because, due to changes at the nasal mucous membrane, dacryocystorhinostomy can not be performed.

The lacrimal sac can be accessed through the incision that starts at 6 to 8 mm medially from the medial corner of the eye, under the medial ligament, and stretches 2-3 cm downward, with a slight lateral inclination (Figure 2). After removing the lacrimal sac it is immediately necessary to conduct a sillicone tube through the lacrimal canaliculi into the nasolacrimal duct. In cases of malignant tumors of the lacrimal sac, particularly the advanced ones, most often it is required to perform exenteration of the orbit with removal of the medial orbital wall.

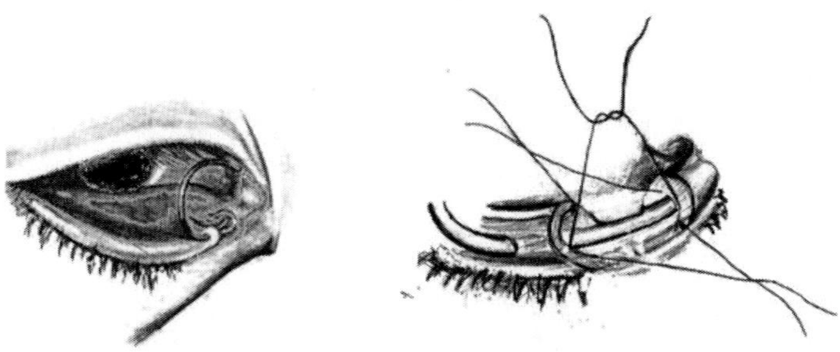

Figure 1. The establishment of continuity of the lacrimal canaliculi after injury or excision of the change on the ductules. A silicone tube is placed into the canaliculi and over it the ends of the ductules have been attached together and stitched with three sutures (7-0 or 8-0).

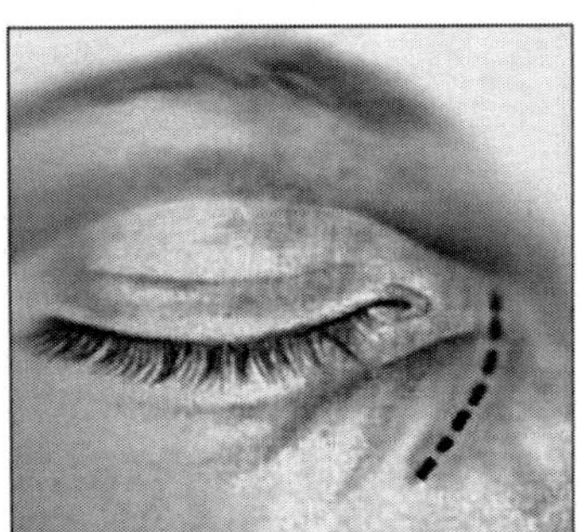

Figure 2. Access to the lacrimal sac through the incision of the skin, the subcutaneous tissue and the periosteum in the area of the medial eye corner.

Traumatic and congenital obstructions of the nasolacrimal canal, for the purpose of establishing the lacrimal drainage into the nose, require a somewhat complex operation – dacryocystorhinostomy [2, 3, 4, 6, 8]. This operation can be performed undre local or total anesthesia. By making an incision through the skin, the subcutaneous tissue and the periosteum, in the area of the medial eye corner (Figure 2), the frontal process of the maxilla and the lacrimal bone are reached. In the course of this incision the angular blood vessels often get injured, and they should be tied off or burnt. The lacrimal sac should be identified and, with deperiosting of the anterior lacrimal crest and the lacrimal fossa, it should be lifted from the fossa. By a round borer or a small instrument for breaking the bones, the bone in front of and behind the lacrimal-maxillary suture should be removed, i.e., almost the entire bone of the lacrimal fossa, the anterior lacrimal crest and a part of the frontal process of the maxilla in front of the anterior crest (Figure 3). In the course of this procedure and during deperiostisation of this region it is necessary to preserve the insertion of the medial ligament. After removing the bone, incision is made on the lacrimal sac and on the nasal mucous membrane for the purpose of forming suitable flaps that are stitched so as to establish continuity between the lacrimal sac and the nasal cavity (Figures 4, 5). Before stitching those flaps a sillicone tube should be placed that shall connect the lacrimal ducts and the nasal cavity. This tube shall prevent the occurrence of a scarred obstruction of a surgically formed lacrimal drainage system in the course of healing of the flaps of the lacrimal sac and the nasal mucous membrane. After stitching the flaps of the lacrimal sac and the nasal mucous membrane, the soft tissues are returned to their position and stitched in a usual manner. After the completed surgery, the patient should be advised to refrain from blowing nose for approximately a ten-day period. If flaps cannot be formed due to the significant changes on the lacrimal sac and a stitch cannot be made with the nasal mucous membrane, then the mucous membrane shall be removed from the point where the flaps and the sutures are usually made. A sillicone tube is inserted from the lacrimal canaliculi through the bony opening in the region of the lacrimal fossa and through the mentioned opening on the nasal mucous membrane into the medium nasal canal. It should be fixed as appropriate onto the nasal mucous membrane to prevent it from falling off. This tube allows the lacrimal canaliculi discharge into the nose through the created fistula. The procedure described is called canaliculorhinostomy or canaliculo-dacryocystorhinostomy [1, 4, 5, 6].

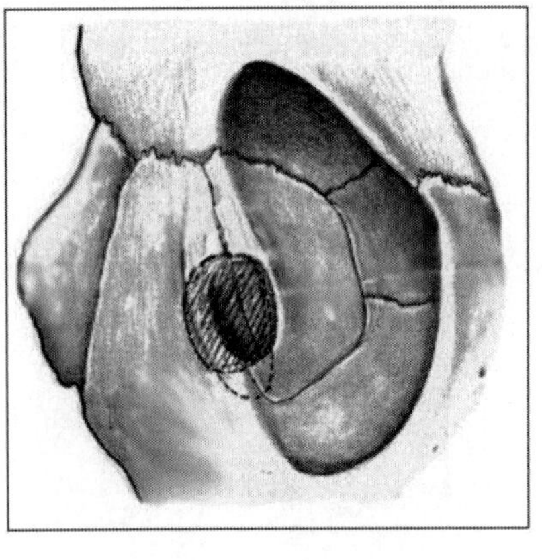

Figure 3. The removal of the bone in the region of the lacrimal fossa for the purpose of introducing dacryocystorhinostomy.

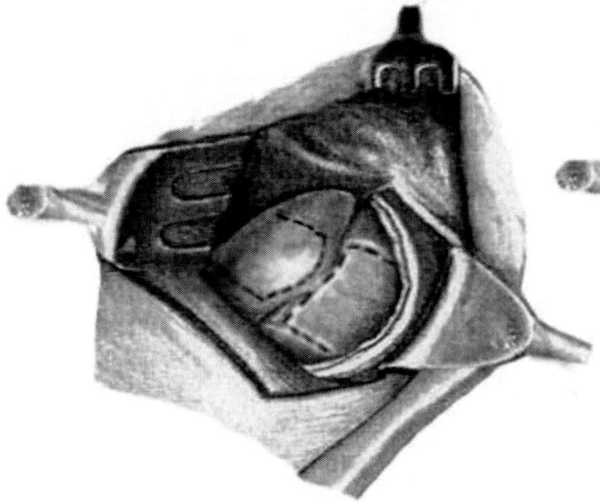

A

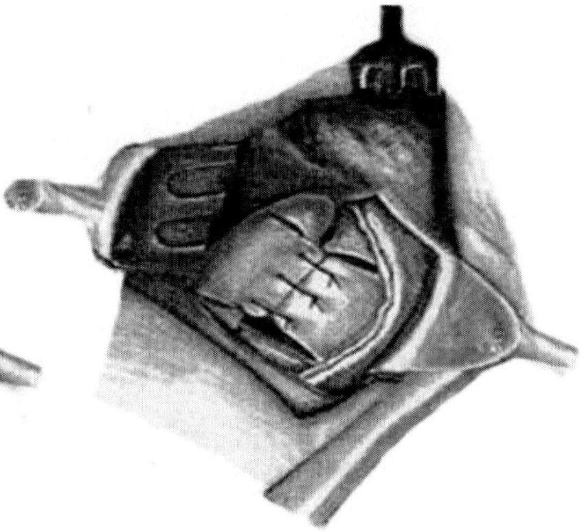

B

Figure 4. A. Incisions on the nasal mucous membrane and the lacrimal sac for the purpose of formation of flaps for establishing dacryocystorhinostomy. B. Stitching of the nasal mucous membrane flaps and the lacrimal sac flaps – establishing dacryocystorhinostomy. First the posterior flaps of the nasal mucous membrane and the lacrimal sac are stitched. Then a silicone tube is inserted up to the nasal cavity, and then the anterior flaps are stitched.

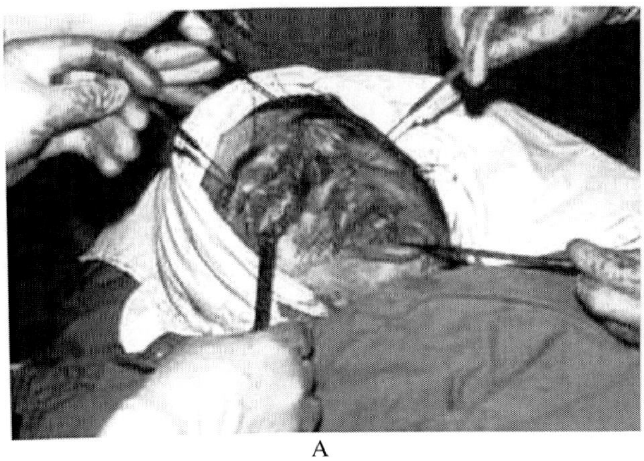

A

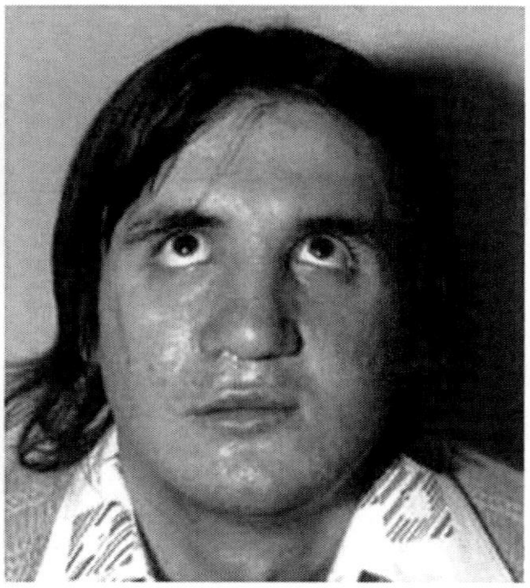

B

Figure 5. A. Patient with a multiple fracture of the facial bones and the nose avulsion. B. The same patient one year after the reposition of the facial bones, the bilateral reconstruction of the orbital floor and the nose reconstruction. In the post-operative period, due to a chronic purulent inflammation of the lacrimal sac caused by the obstruction of the nasolacrimal duct, a dacryocystorhinostomy was performed.

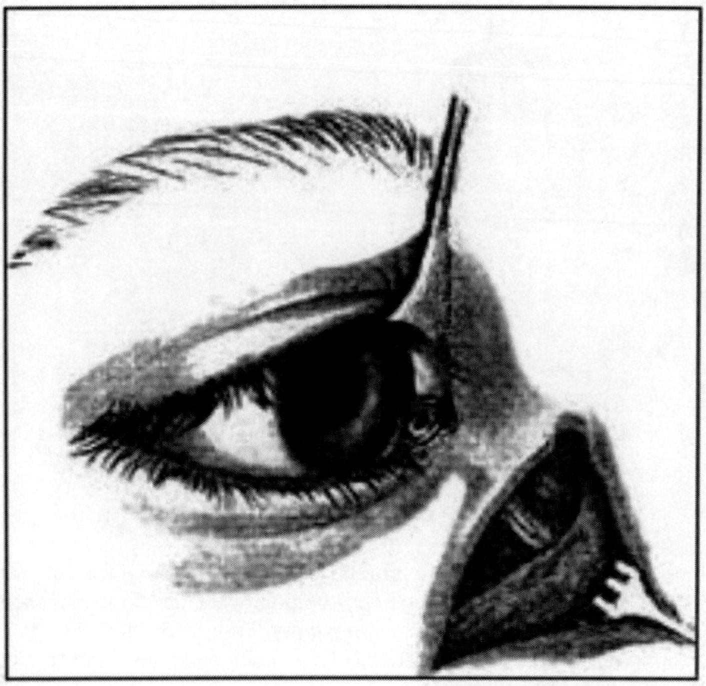

Figure 6. For the purposes of the conjunctivo (dacryo)rhinostmy, the silicone tube has been inserted up to the nasal cavum through the spot where the caruncle once stood, through the lacrimal sac and through the opening on the bone of the lacrimal fossa and the nasal mucous membrane.

In cases of congenital absence of the lacrimal canaliculi or in cases when, due to injuries or operations, their passability cannot be established, it is necessary to form a fistula surgically that will connect the conjunctival space with the nose. This procedure is called conjunctivodacryocystorhinostomy [2, 4, 5, 6]. If there is no lacrimal sac, then a fistula is formed between the conjunctival space and the nose and this procedure is called conjunctivorhinostomy. The approach for these surgical procedures is the same as for dacryocystorhinostomy. In the same manner an opening is made on the bone in the region of the lacrimal fossa. If there is a lacrimal sac, but the tears cannot pass into the nose, communication and the passability of tears to the nasal cavity are established in the same manner as in dacryocystorhinostomy. In order to establish communication of the conjunctival space to the lacrimal sac or the nasal cavity, the excision of the caruncle must be performed, and then, by a sharp preparation, through the place where the caruncle was, to reach the lacrimal sac, i.e., the opening on the bone which has been previously made in the area of the lacrimal fossa. From the place where the caruncle once existed the tube is inserted (of silicone, glass or polyethylene) into the middle nasal meatus through the lacrimal sac (if there is one), through the opening on the bone at the lacrimal fossa level (same opening as for dacryocystorhinostomy) and through the opening on the nasal mucous membrane (same opening as for canaliculorhinostomy). The tube is fixed onto the nasal mucous membrane in a certain manner. This tube must occasionally be taken out and cleaned.

5.4. Patients and Surgical Therapy Results

In fife patients, the suture of the lacrimal canaliculi was performed over a silicone tube after injury. In seven patients, under general anesthesia, dacryocystorhinostomy was performed in a usual manner because of the obstruction of the nasolacrimal duct (Figure 6). In one patient canaliculo-dacryocystorhinostomy was performed and conjunctivodacryocystorhinostomy in another one. With exception of three cases (postoperative strictures) good or satisfactory results were achieved in all patients.

Conclusion

The entire surgery of the lacrimal apparatus – the lacrimal gland, the lacrimal canaliculi, the lacrimal sac and the nasolacrimal duct – requires the application of diverse surgical methods and techniques. Due to a narrow lumen of the lacrimal excretory system, potential post-operative fibrosis and stricture, it is not always possible to achieve satisfactory results. Nevertheless, with a good training in surgical procedures and techniques, patience and adequate post-operative treatment, the satisfactory result should be a norm. No patient should be left with a permanent discomfort – a lifetime lacrimation.

References

[1] Angrist R. C., Dortzbach R. K., Silicone intubation for partial and total nasolacrimal duct obstruction in adults, *Ophthal. Plast. Reconstr. Surg.* 1: 51 -54.

[2] Converse J. M., Smith B., Defects in lacrimal system, in: Converse J. M., Reconstructive Plastic Surgery, Vol II, Saunders, Philadelphia, 1977.

[3] Dortzbach R. K., Dacryocystorhinostomy, *Trans. Am. Acad. Ophthalmol. Otol.* 85: 1267 -1270, 1978.

[4] Jones L. T., Woobing J. L., Surgery of the eyelids and lacrimal system, Birmingham, Ala: Aesculapius, 1976.

[5] Lauring L., Silicone intubation of the lacrimal system, *Am. Ophthalmol.* 8: 489 – 498, 1976.

[6] Lemke B. N., Della Rocca R. C., Surgery of the eyelids & orbits, Prentice – *Hall International*, 1990.

[7] Rončević R., Rončević D., Surgical treatment of severe dysthyroid exophthalmos-long term results, *J. Craniomaxillofac. Surg.* 23: 355 – 362, 1995.

[8] Zolli C. L., Shannon G. M., Dacryocystorhinostomy: A review of 119 cases, *Ophthalmic Surg.* 13: 905 – 910, 1982.

Chapter 6

Surgery of Congenital Orbital Malformations

6.1. Introduction

Congenital malformations of the craniofacial region occur in approximately 42 out of 1000 newborns [6]. Since the orbit represents the central part of the craniofacial region, the congenital malformations of the orbit are usually a part of a more complex syndrome that affects the bones of the skull and the face, i.e., the craniofacial region.

The causes of orbital malformations may be:

- Aplasia or hypoplasia of the eye or the brain,
- various facial clefts,
- premature synostosis of the cranial and facial bones that cause craniosynostosis (craniostenosis) or various syndroms of craniofacial synostosis

These pathological conditions result in various malformations of the orbit, such as aplasia or hypoplasia, absence of the part of the orbit, orbital dystopia, hypertelorism or formation of the short and shallow orbits. All these anomalies significantly affect development and function of the eye and its adnexa. A certain percentage of people who have normal anatomic structures of the cranial and facial skeleton have somewhat shallower and shorter orbits, manifested by a visible eye protrusion, the eyes are "big," similar to patients with exophthalmos in cases of dysthyroid ophthalmopathy [16].

Thanks to development of craniofacial surgery, even some monstrous deformities of the cranial and facial skeleton, as well as the orbit, can be brought into an acceptable state.

6.2. Correction of "Big Eyes" in People with Shallow and Short Orbits

The orbit has the shape of a modified cone or a pyramid. The length of the anterioposterior, longitudinal axis is about 45 mm [1, 5, 8, 9, 16, 17]. The bulbar part of the orbital floor is more or less concave, while the retrobulbar part is slightly convex [1, 5, 8, 9, 16, 17]. In people with "big eyes"the bulbar part of the orbital floor is flat, or even slightly convex, and the retrobulbar part of the orbit is significantly convex [8, 16, 17]. If, along with that, the anteroposterior diameter of the orbit is shorter, then the orbital volume is significantly reduced. That is why the eye is positioned more outside the orbit than in people with a normal orbital shape and volume. "Big eyes" due to somewhat shallower and shorter orbits, in people with normal anatomic structures of the face and the skull, are seen very rarely. They are symmetrically "big", with normal movement and without functional disturbances. "Big eyes" are only aesthetic failure. (Figures 1, 2).

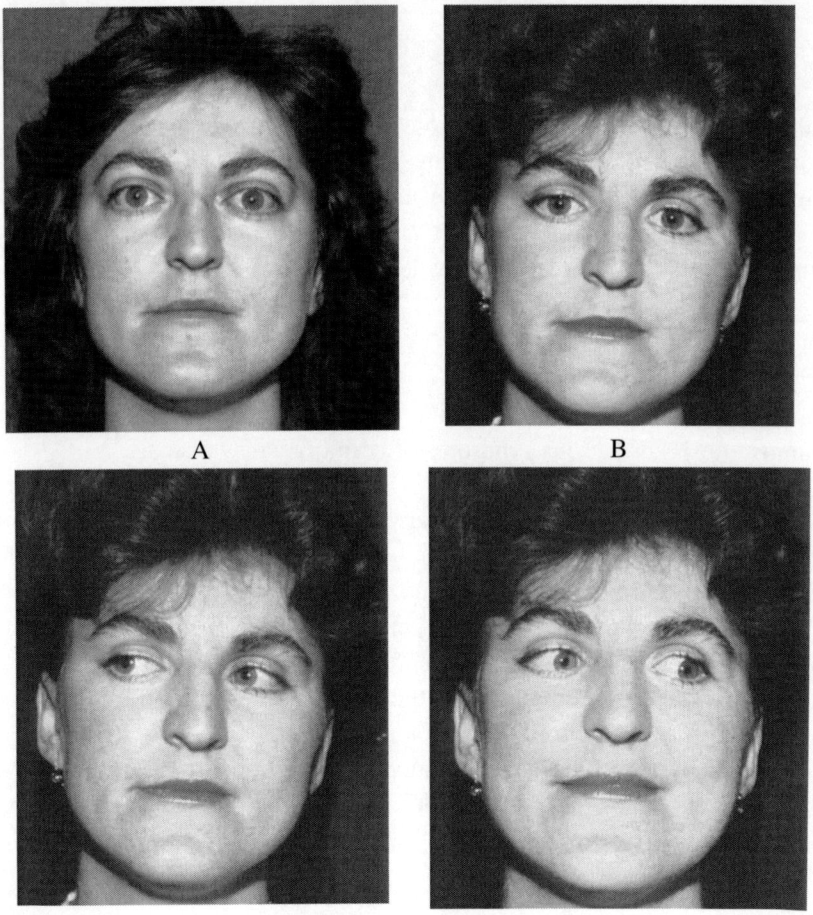

A B C D

Figure 1. A. Pre-operative look of a twenty-seven-year-old patient with "big eyes" (exophthalmos 25 mm). B. The patient three months after the operation. C. Look right.
D-Look left.

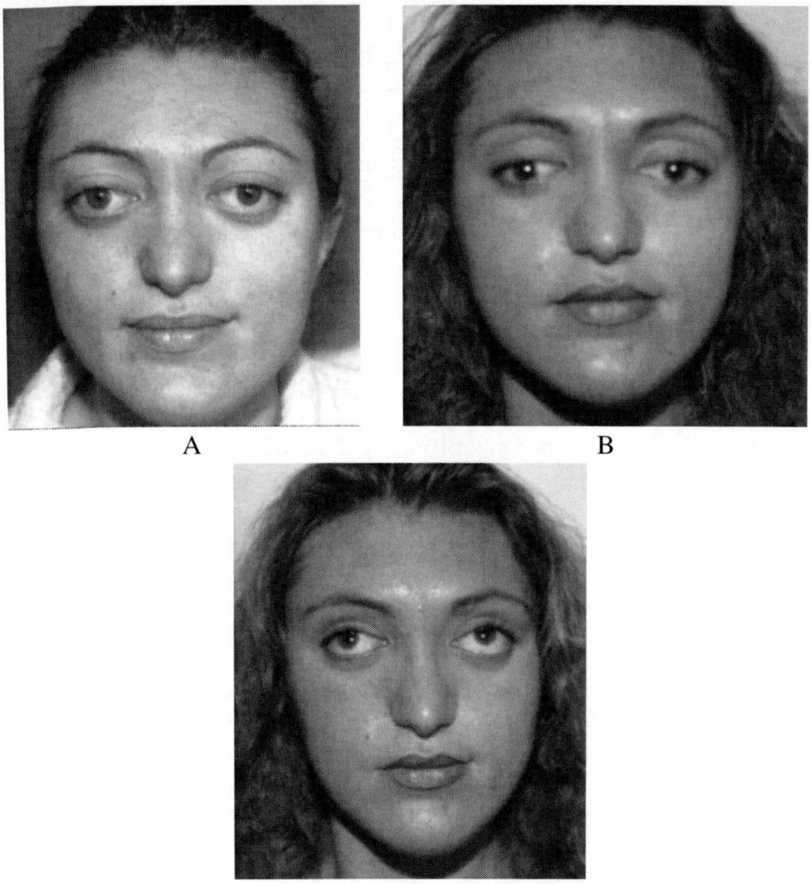

A B

C

Figure 2. A. Preoperative look of a twenty year old patient with "big eyes" (exophthalmos 25 mm) and strabismus. B. The patient three months after the operation. Strabismus is less evident and there is no double vision. C. Look upwards.

The final diagnosis of the "big eyes" is obtained after a detailed endocrinological and ophthalmological examination, and after a CT image and orbital echography. In this manner, a latent or slight dysthyroid exophthalmos, retrobulbar tumor or any pathological process of the orbit are excluded.

The surgical procedure starts with a subciliary incision on the lower eyelid. Through this incision, the infraorbital margin is reached in a usual manner. After the completed incision of the periosteum along the infraorbital margin, the entire orbital floor is explored, the periorbital and orbital fat tissue is removed, and then by a small chisel and hemostat the retrobulbar part of the orbital floor is also removed. This means that the anterior, bulbar part of the orbital floor, on which the eye lies, must remain intact so that the eye will not fall towards the maxillary sinus. In the course of the removal of the retrobulbar part of the orbital floor the injury of the infraorbital nerve must be avoided. This is achieved by removing bone on either side and then freeing the nerve. The injury of the lower extraocular muscles must also be avoided, as well as a major injury of the maxillary sinus mucosa. Small perforations of the sinus mucosa are of no importance. During removal of the retrobulbar part of the orbital floor, in order to avoid injury of the optic nerve, should not enter into the region of optic nerve opening. After chemostasis, the eyelid wound is stitched in a usual manner. In a single operative act the same surgical procedure is performed on both orbits. The following day after the surgery the patient starts with exercises of the eye movement in all directions, especially upwards, so that the postoperative scar around extraocular muscles would not restrict their function, which may result in the occurrence of double vision.

With described surgical treatment the relations of the orbit are changed, similary to the cases of blowout fractures of the orbital floor, that is, the volume of the orbit is significantly increased The increase of the orbital volume allows a deeper retraction of the eye into the orbit, which results in the eye becoming "smaller." With removal of the orbital fat tissue the additional space for the eye is provided. The operation must be performed with precision, with symmetrical removal of the fat tissue and the orbital bones on both sides. Naturally, care should be taken not to remove too much of the bone because it may result in enophthalmos, particularly if during the operation the orbital fat tissue has also been removed. If this operation is performed with precision, there is no risk for the eyesight and the normal eye function is preserved (Figures 1, 2).

In cases of less evident "big eyes," it is possible to obtain a satisfactory correction of the eye position by removing orbital fat tissue without removal of the part of the orbital floor.

6.3. Orbital Hypoplasia and Surgical Treatment

Development of the orbit is related to development of the eye. In cases of primary anophthalmos or microophthalmos the orbit cannot be developed – it remains too small. Such a condition is called orbital hypoplasia or microorbitism. The loss of an eye in early childhood caused by an injury or enucleation because of a tumor also results in orbital hypoplasia, particularly if being post-operatively subjected to the irradiation therapy [7, 14] (Figure 3). The orbital hypoplasia is followed by hypoplasia of the periorbital bony and soft structures, i.e., hypoplasia of the supraorbital, zygomatic and infraorbital region. Sometimes hemifacial hypoplasia can be observed [2] (Figure 3).

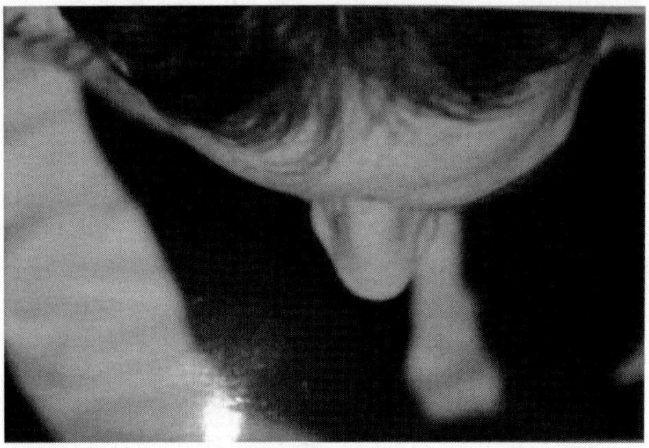

Figure 3. The condition after enucleation and iradiation tharapy in early childhood. Very evident hypolasia of the orbit, supraorbital, zygomatic and infraorbital regions with hemifacial hypoplasia.

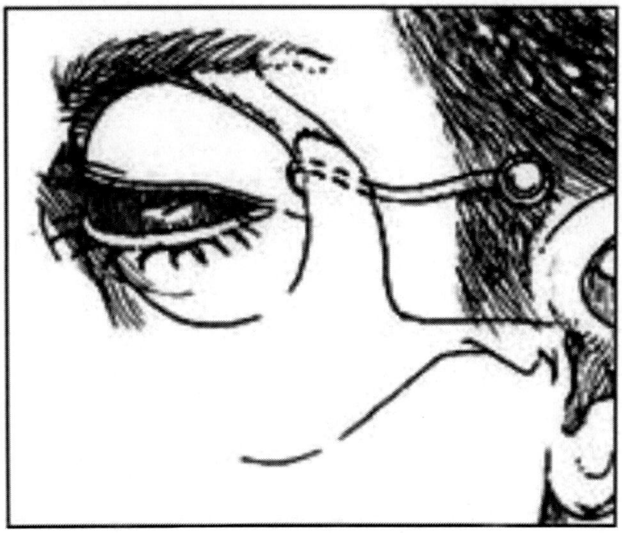

Figure 4. Intraorbital expander has been inserted into the orbit subperiostally. The tube for filling the expander has been pulled into the temporal region through the opening on the lateral orbital wall. At the beginning of the tube there is a valve through which the expander is filled.

Correction of orbital hypoplasia should be initiated as soon as possible. Certain results can be achieved by application of a series of adequate eye prothesis (getting larger and larger) [2]. This treatment starts in early childhood and continues through puberty. Good adaptation of the prothesis, simulating the eye, often requires performance of a major or minor corrective procedure on the eyelids and the conjunctival sac.

Better results can be achieved by application of the intraorbital tissue expanders [2]. By making a semi-circular incision in the temporal region, in the hairy part, the lateral orbital wall is explored and a minor opening is made on it. The expander is placed subperiostally into the orbit and through the opening on the lateral orbital wall the tube for filling the expander is pulled into the temporal region. At the beginning of the tube a valve is located through which the expander is filled (Figure 4). The expander is being gradually filled with physiological solution over the period of three months. After the expansion has been completed, an adequate eye prothesis is inserted into the orbit. However, the eyelids and the conjunctival sac must previously be reconstructed. The best results can be achieved if the orbital expansion has been initiated at an early age, i.e., six to eight weeks after a child has been born. After the 25th week from birth the effect of expansion becomes significantly reduced [3]. A major expansion effect should not be expected in cases when the irradiation therapy of the orbit has been conducted [2].

In cases of microorbitism, when early orbital expansion has not been conducted or when such early expansion did not give a satisfactory result, it is possible to enlarge the orbit by performing osteotomy of its walls. It is a complex surgical procedure requiring excellent knowledge of craniofacial surgery [10]. By a coronal incision in the hairy part of the frontal and temporal regions all soft tissues are separeted from bone up to the supraorbital margins, with exploring those margins. A bilateral exploration is required for the purpose of comparing the outcome of the surgery. A subciliary incision on the lower eyelid allows exploration of the infraorbital margin and the orbital floor on the side where hypoplasia is located.

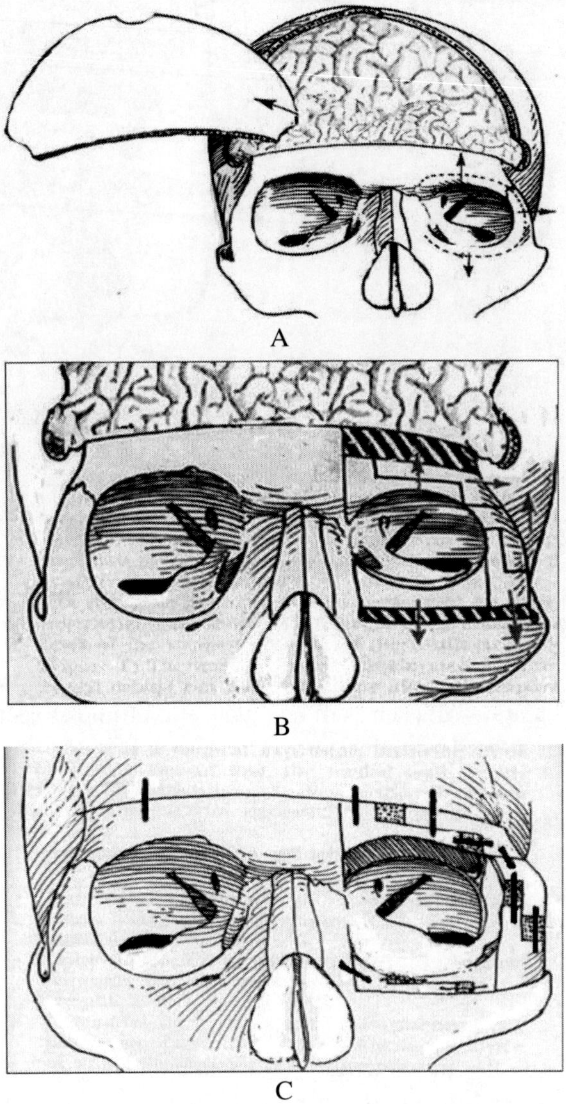

Figure 5. Surgical enlargement of anophthalmic socket by Marchac. A- Fontal craniotomy and directions of walls transposition of the hypoplastic orbit B. Osteotomic incisions on the orbit: parts of bones have been removed supraorbitally and infraorbitally in the form of a horizontal strip (marked). C. Osteotomized fragments of the orbit have been moved towards the periphery to a new position. This is provided by previous removal of the bone in the supraorbital and the infraorbital region. The bony fragments are fixed by mini/micro plates to the surrounding bone. A bone defect between the osteotomized fragments of the bone has been filled by parts of the bone which has previously been removed in the supraorbital and the infraorbital region.

Frontal craniotomy is performed by a neurosurgical technique (Figure 5A). Its lower horizontal line is one centimeter above the level of the supraorbital margin on the healthy, undamaged side (Figure 5A). The soft tissues with the temporal muscle are separated on the hypoplastic side from the lateral margin and the lateral orbital wall. The base of the brain is lifted from the orbital roof through the "window"on the frontal bone for the purpose of approaching the orbit from the cranial, brain side. A part of the frontal bone is removed on the hypoplastic side above the supraorbital margin, along the supraorbital margin, in the width required for elevation of the supraorbital margin (Figure 5B). This is followed by the osteotomy of the superior, inferior and lateral orbital margin, with the anterior part of the corresponding orbital walls. Osteotomy is performed by a small electric saw or a borer with a small diameter. In order to lower the inferior and the lateral margin with the part of the corresponding wall it is necessary to cut a horizontal strip in the infraorbital region of the maxilla and of the zygomatic bone in the width required for lowering the inferior and the lateral orbital margin (Figure 5B).

After osteotomy has been completed the fragments of the orbital margins with the part of the corresponding orbital wall are placed into a new position, which is provided by a previous removal of the part of the frontal and the zygomatic bone, and the maxilla (Figure 5C). Those fragments are fixed to the surrounding bones by wire ligatures or by mini i.e., microplates. The parts of the bones removed from the supraorbital or the infraorbital region are previously placed in the space in which the bone fragments do not touch each other (Figure 5C).

The orbit can be significantly enlarged by using the method described thus making it symmetrical to the opposite side. The frontal bone fragment has restored its original position and it has been fixed to the surrounding bones by wire ligatures or by micro i.e., miniplates. The soft tissues are also returned to their original position and stitched in a usual manner. Lateral canthopexy is also required. In the course of osteotomy of the inferior margin and the orbital floor the infraorbital nerve must be preserved. Since the teeth buds have been positioned quite high, they can be demaged during the removal of the horizontal strip of the bone in the infraorbital region. That is why a proper roentgenological diagnosis is required in the pre-operative period so that the position of the teeth buds could be determined. In the course of the operation described, in the same act, the remains of the eye must be removed and the conjunctival sac must be enlarged by the application of a skin or mucous free transplant of partial thickness. The correction of the eyelids must be performed in the same or the following surgical procedure. A good eye prothesis requires a successful previously conducted reconstruction of the orbit, the conjunctival sac and the eyelids.

6.4. Orbital Malformations Caused by Facial Cleft and Their Treatment

The facial clefts, although very rare, can appear on any part of the face. The cause of the clefts, debated in several theories, has not been fully understood. The most widely accepted classification of clefts was made by Tessier in 1976 [21]: fifteen clefts numbered 0 to 14 (Figure 6). All these clefts pass through the orbit or are in its immediate vicinity and inevitably cause various orbital deformities, most often a partial defect of soft and bony tissues (Figures 7, 8, 9), hypertelorism or orbital dystopia. In cases of defects of the soft and bony tissues of the face and the orbit, first requirement is that the soft tissues be reconstructed by various surgical procedures applying local or distant skin, fascial or musculo-cutaneous flaps (Figure 7), i.e., by applying the flaps transferred by a microsurgical anastomosis. In the same or following surgical act, the absence of a part of the orbit and the surrounding structures shall be reconstructed by various surgical methods using the bones of the skull, the hip, the scapula or the rib cartilage [4, 6, 11, 13, 15, 18, 19] (Figures 7, 8, 9).

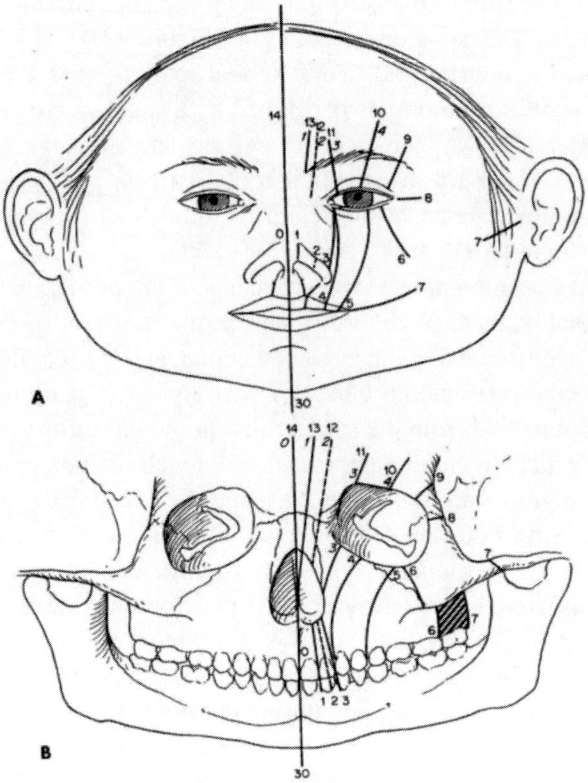

Figure 6. Tessier classification of facial clefts (Tessier P.: Anatomical classification of facial, cranio-facial and lateral clefts, J. Maxullofac. Surge 4:69-92,1976) A. place of a facial cleft, B. place of the cleft on the facial skeleton.

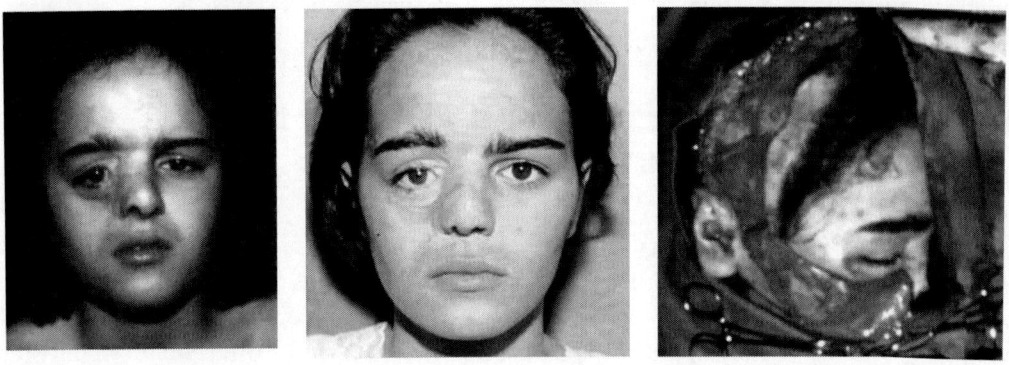

A B C

Figure 7. A, B. The condition after the correction of the complete cleft No.3 and 4. Facial tissues have been reconstructed, as well as the eyelids, half of the nose, the upper lip, the anterior part of the maxilla, the medial orbital wall, the orbital floor and the infraorbital margin. The eye has been lifted for 8 mm. C. one of the reconstructive details – use of pericranial flap.

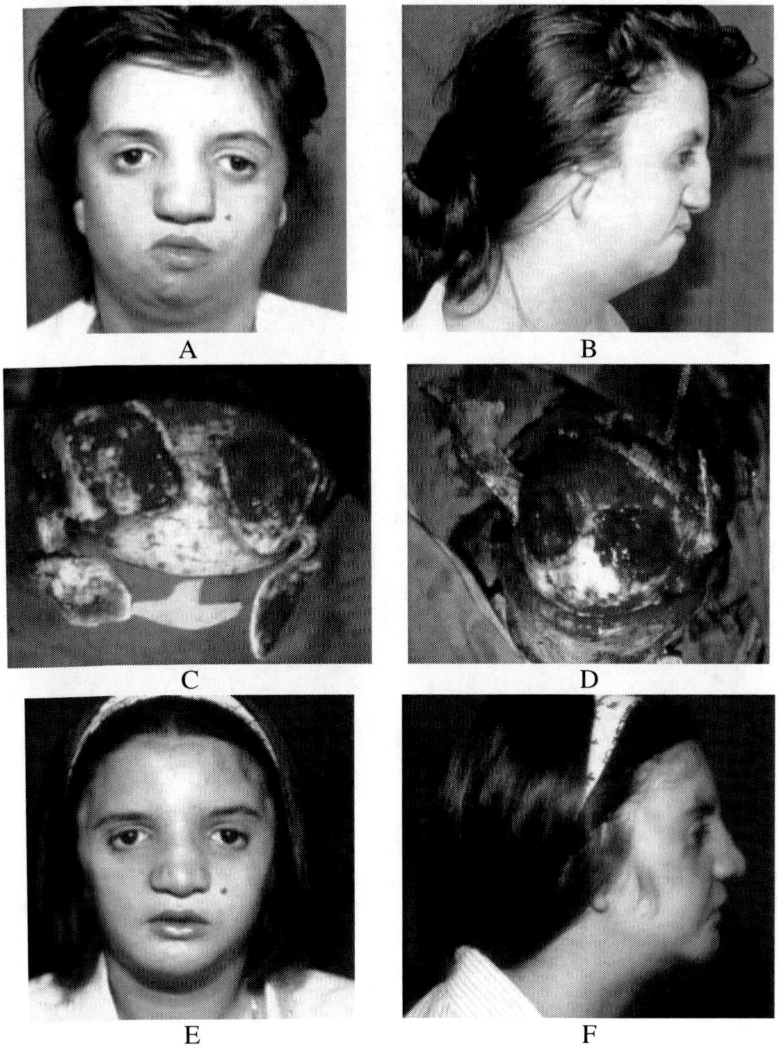

Figure 8. A, B. Treacher Collins' syndrome (clefts 6, 7 and 8): the lack of the zygomatic bone and the infraorbital margin, colobom on the lower eyelids, the absence of eyelashes on the medial part of the lower eyelids, microtia, hypoplasia of jaws with nasal deformity. C. Osteopericranial flap – vascularized parietal bone on the pedicle of the pericranium, i.e., on the pedicle of the temporal superficial artery and vein. D. Vascularized bone has been moved bilaterally, through the subcutaneous tunnel, into the zygomatico – infraorbital region. The additional pericranial flap has been lifted bilaterally. These flaps have been folded, duplicated and used for correcting, filling the temporal region. E, F. The same patient two years after the operation. The upper and the lower jaw have been moved frontward after an adequate osteotomy, the zygomatico-infraorbital part with the inferior orbital margin has been corrected bilaterally by using osteopericranial flaps. The temporal region has been filled bilaterally by a duplicated pericranial flap. Rhinoplasty has been performed within the same procedure.

In cases of hypertelorism or orbital dystopia, in order to correct the malformation, complex craniofacial surgical procedures must be applied, which shall be described in the following pages.

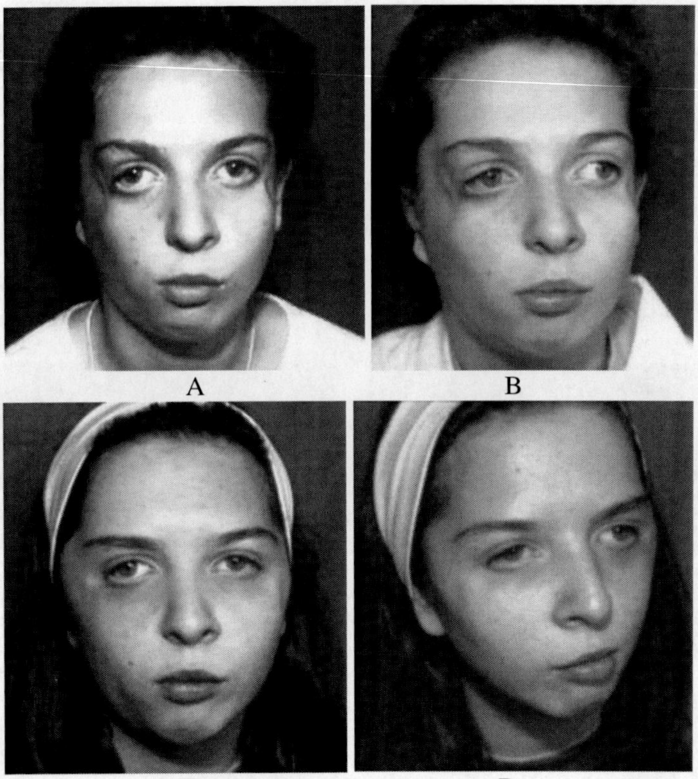

A B C D

Figure 9. A, B. Pre-operative look of the patient with Treacher Collins syndrome: the absence of the lateral orbital wall bilaterally, hypoplasia of the temporal and the zygomatic bone bilaterally, coloboma of the lower eyelids and the absence of eyelashes on the medial part of the lower eyelids. C, D. The same patient one year after the operation. The zygomatico-temporal region has been corrected bilaterally by the osteopericranial flaps – the parietal bone which has been transferred to the zygomatico-temporal region on the pericranial flap, i.e., on temporal blood vessels.

A relatively frequent type of a facial cleft, with changes on the orbit and the eyelids, is mandibulofacial dysostosis, which is most often referred to as Treacher Collins' (Francheschetti) syndrome (Figures. 8, 9). It is a complex syndrome with three clefts – 6, 7 and 8. The cleft is located in the maxillozygomatic, the temporozygomatic and the frontozygomatic suture. The consequence of these clefts is the absence of the zygomatic bone and the zygomatic arch, with the corresponding part of the orbital floor, the absence of the lateral orbital margin, the lower eyelid coloboma, the absence of eyelashes on the medial two-thirds of the lower eyelid, dystopia of the lateral corner of the eye, which gives an antimongolian look, and hypoplasia of the temporal and the masseteric muscle. In persons with this syndrome the jaws are underdeveloped, with irregular teeth occlusion. For correcting this complex anomaly the application of complex craniofacial procedure is required [4, 6, 12, 15, 18, 19] (Figures 8, 9).

In some cases of progressive hemifacial atrophy – Romberg's disease, atrophy of the infraorbital region and the infraorbital margin occur, in addition to an evident enophthalmos due to the atrophy of the orbital fat tissue. In such cases correction of the infraorbital region and correction of the enophthalmos are indicated, and are performed similarly to corrections in posttraumatic enophthalmos [17, 19] (Figures 10, 11).

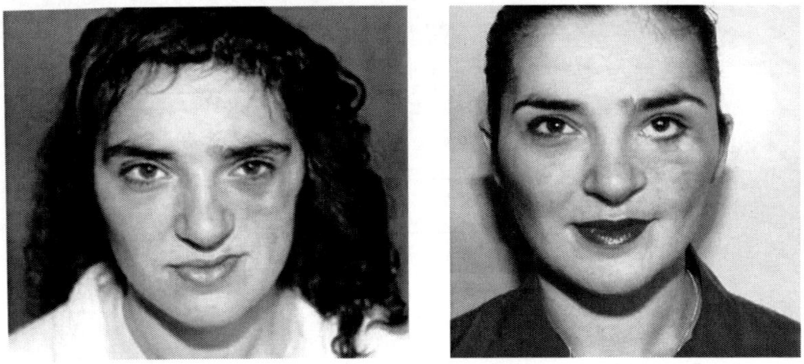

A B

Figure 10. A. The patient with Romberg's disease – atrophy and deformity of the left side of the face, especially of the infraorbital region, with enophthalmos due to the orbital fat atrophy. B. The condition after the operation. The correction of the infraorbital region has been made by a duplicated, pericranial flap. Enophthalmos and infraorbital margin have been corrected by calvarial bone graft. Because of the basic disease the lower eyelid is atrophic and atonic. The patient still has not decided to undergo this minor correction.

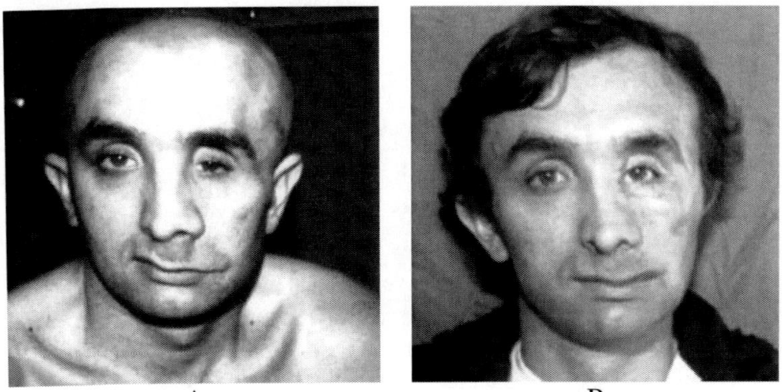

A B

Figure 11. A. Romerg's disease with enophtalmos due to orbital fat atrophy and neurofibromatosis of face, nose, lips and palate. B. The condition one year aftre the insertion of duplicate pericranial flap into subcutaneous space of the face, correction of neurofibromatosis and correction of enophthalmos using a piece of calvarial bone.

6.5. Orbital Malformations Caused by Premature Synostosis of Cranial and Facial Bones and Their Treatment

Premature synostosis of the cranial bones – craniostenosis – may occur at one or more cranial sutures, with various deformities of the skull and the orbit [4, 6, 11, 12, 13, 20]. Disorders of development of the skull often lead to increase in the intracranial pressure, which may cause disorders of psychomotor development, as well as various vision disorders. All craniosynostoses (craniostenoses) may be classifed in five groups:

- *Scaphocephaly* – synostosis of the sagittal suture. The skull is elongated in the sagital direction, and flattened in the transversal direction.
- *Brachycephaly* – bilateral synostosis in the coronal suture. The skull is short in the sagittal direction, and wide in the transversal direction.
- *Plagiocephaly* – unilateral coronal synostosis, the forehead is asymmetric, not developed on the side affected by synostosis. The eyebrow and the superior orbital margin are in retrusion and slightly elevated. The opposite side of the forehead is developed normally, the forehead is protruded, whereas the orbit has a major or minor inferolateral dystopia (Figure 12);
- *Trigonocephaly* – synostosis of the frontal, metopic suture. The anterior cranial fossa and the forehead are triangularly deformed, so the forehead in the central line is boat-shaped; the orbits have been moved medially, and there is hypotelorism.
- *Multiple synostoses,* result in various and very evident cranial deformities, such as turricephaly, oxycephaly etc., with various deformities of the orbit and the eye protrusion.

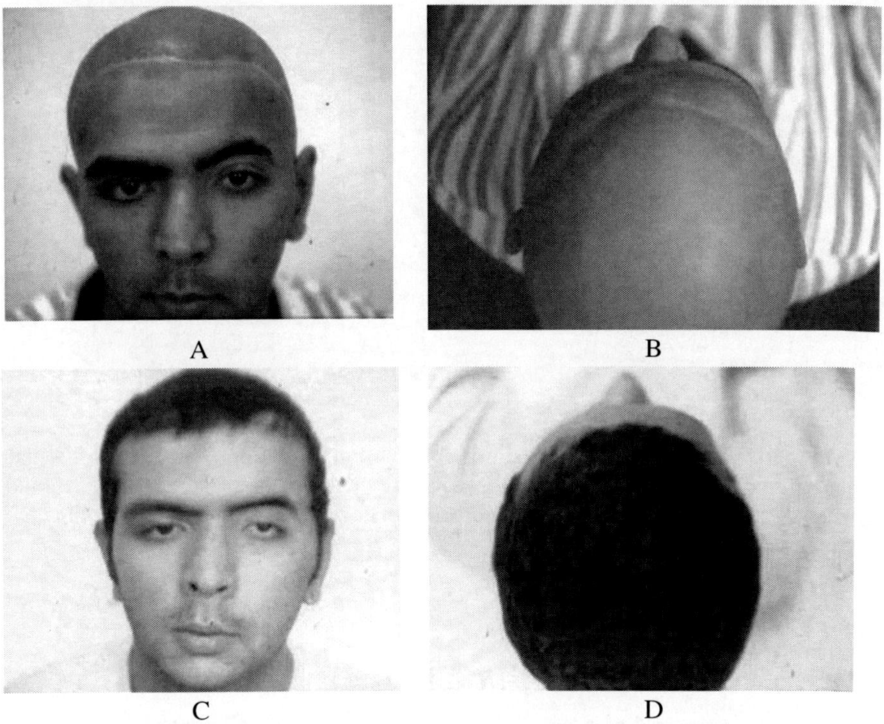

Figure 12. A, B. Plagiocephaly in an adult – the condition after failed correction in a neurosurgical institution. Forehead asymmetry and underdeveloped upper part of the left orbit. C, D. The patient after the operation – correction of the frontal and supraorbital region.

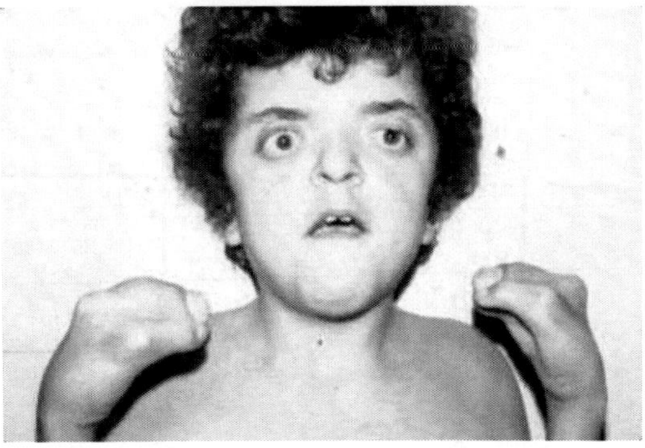

Figure 13. The patient with Apert syndrome – craniofacial synostosis with syndactylia.

The most common syndromes of the craniofacial synostoses are Crouzon syndrome, Apert syndrome and Pfeiffer syndrome. These syndromes are characterized by evident hypoplasia of the middle third of the face with various skull deformities, depending on in which suture the premature synostosis took place, hypertelorism or orbital dystopia and very evident bilateral eye protrusion due to shallow and short orbits. In cases of Crouzon syndrome only craniofacial.synostosis exists. If craniofacial synostosis is accompanied by syndactylia of the hands and feet, it is Apert syndrome (Figure 13). In cases of Pfeiffer syndrome, apart from craniofacial synostosis, the thumbs on the feet are enlarged and significantly detached from the other finger.

Orbital hypertelorism represents a special form of craniofacial deformity. Various prenatal clefts and premature synostoses of cranial and facial structures are the main causes of orbital hypertelorism. Hypertelorism is often caused by meningoencephalocele – congenital brain and meninges herniation through the craniofacial skeleton defect. Large pneumatization, i.e., the width of the ethmoid and the frontal sinuses may also cause hypertelorism. In newborns having normal skulls the distance between the medial orbital walls is 16 mm on average. In normally developed skulls of adults the distance between the medial orbital walls is about 25 mm. The distance from 30 to 34 mm is regarded as the first degree of hypertelorism. The distance from 35 to 40 mm represents the second degree, whereas the distance exceeding 40 mm is the third degree of hypertelorism.

Surgical corrections of cranial and orbital deformities, occurring as the result of premature synostosis of the cranial and facial bones, include comprehensive, complex and complicated surgical procedures which are in the domain of craniofacial surgery, a young surgical discipline that started to develop some forty-five years ago. The creator of this surgery is the famous French surgeon, Paul Tessier (20, 21). It is simply impossible to present all the methods and details of these surgical procedures in a book dealing with orbital surgery, despite the fact that the orbit is most often the center of such operations. That is why only the principles of craniofacial surgery shall be presented in this chapter in order to understand the possibilities and the achievements of such complicated surgical procedures. Using as an example the surgical treatment of hypertelorism, one of the most complex procedures in the domain of craniofacial surgery, it is possible to understand the basic principle of the surgical treatment of cranial and craniofacial stenosis and malformations, which are accompanied by diverse orbital malformations [4, 6, 11, 12, 13, 20].

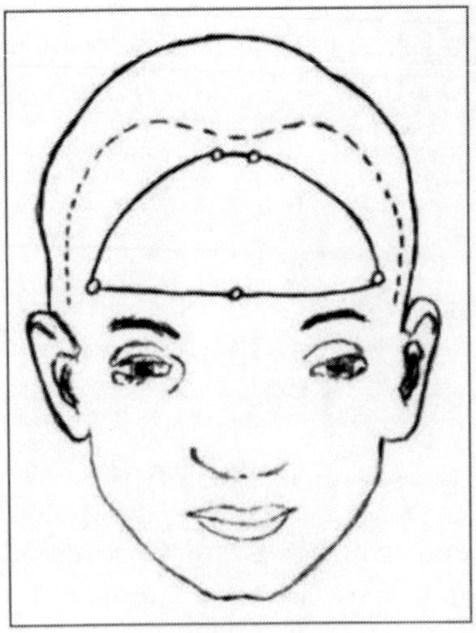

A

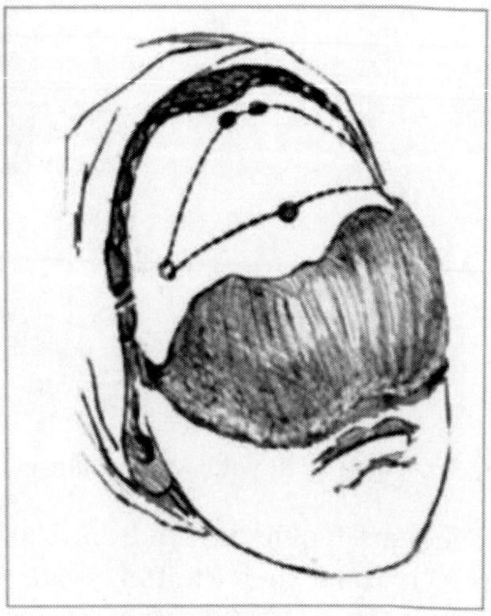

B

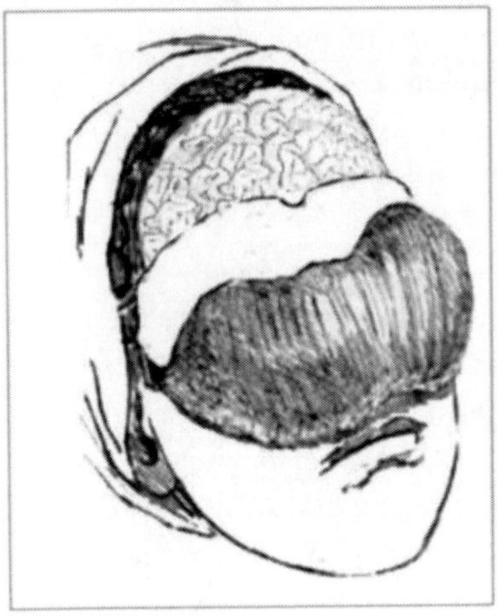

C

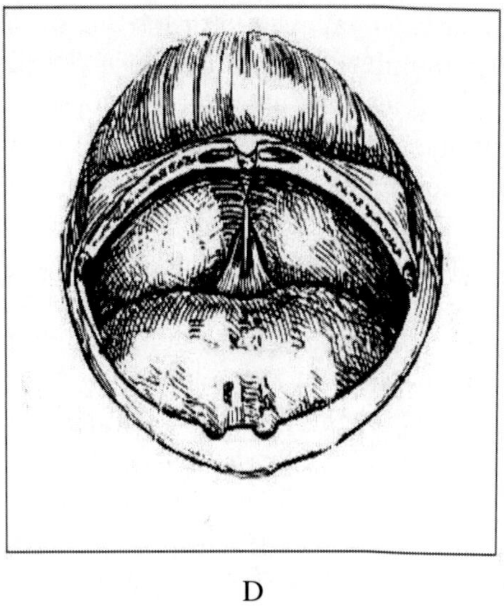

D

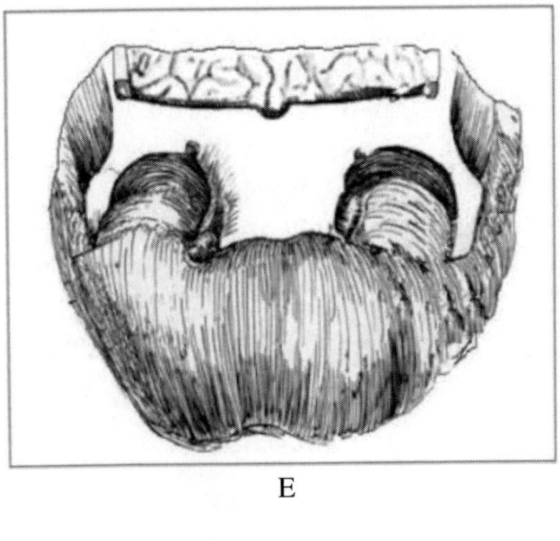

E

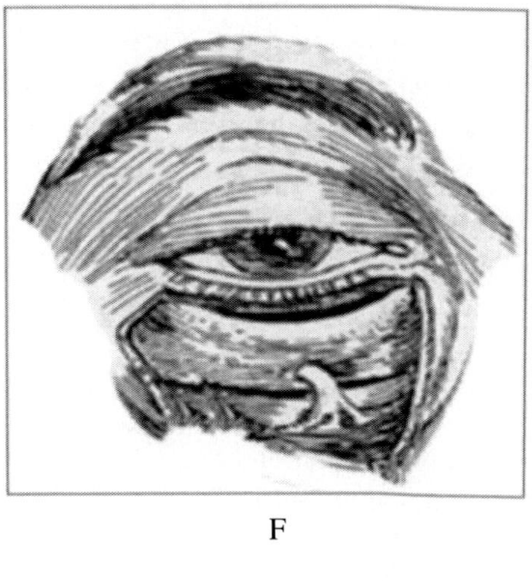

F

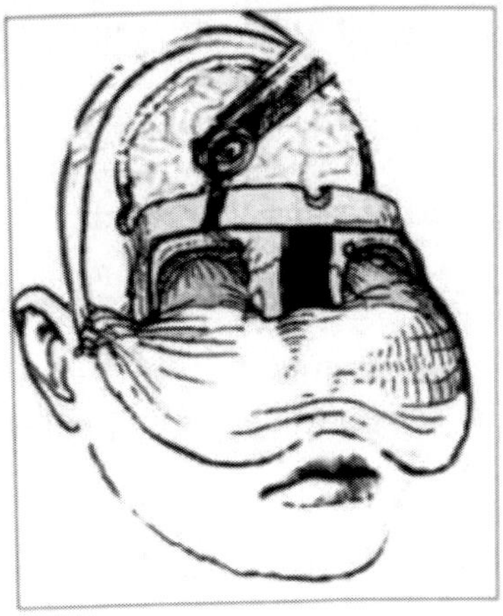

G

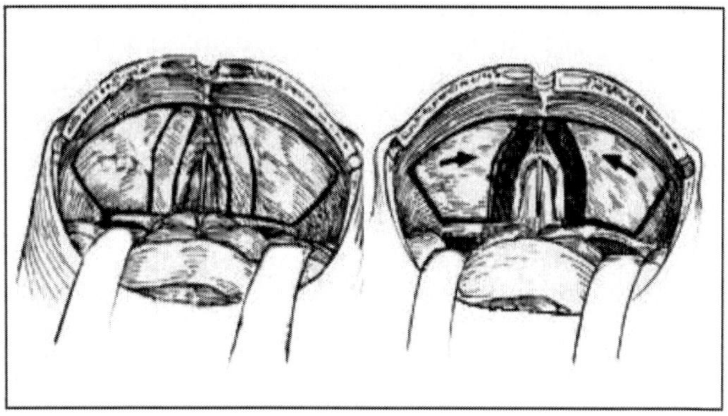

H

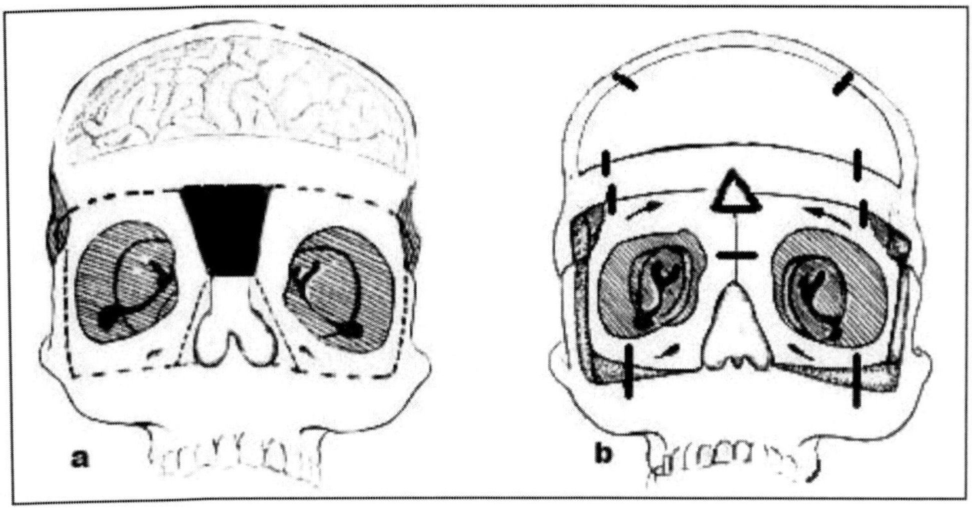

I

Figure 14. A. B. Coronal incision and frontal bone osteotomy. C. A part of the frontal bone has been removed. D. The base of the brain is lifted ofthe skull base and the roof of both orbits E. By deperiosting, the superior, the medial and the lateral orbital walls have been freed from the orbital content deep down up to the fusion of the posterior and the middle third of the orbit. F. The infraorbital part of the maxilla and of the zygomatic bone have been deperiosted, as well as the orbital floor deep down up to the fusion of the posterior and the middle third of the orbit. The infraorbital nerve has been isolated. G. Orbital osteotomy: in order to move the orbits into a new position, the excess of the bone in the medial line must be removed (marked). H. Intracranial osteotomic incisions: in order to move the orbits into a new position, the excess of the bone in front and on both sides of cribriform plate must be removed. Ia. Osteotomy of both orbits has been performed along with the removal of the bone in the medial line, on the nasal crest area and on both sides of the cribriform lamina. Ib. The orbits have been brought into a new position and fixed onto the supraorbital strip of the frontal bone, and also mutually. Into the empty space between the orbits and the surrounding bones the parts of the bone are put which is taken of the outer lamina of the calvaria or the hip. The frontal bone has been put back in its position and fixed to the adjacent bone.

After complete internist (pediatric), neuropsychiatric, ophthalmological, laboratory, radiographic and cephalometric examinations and tests, the plan for surgical procedure is made. For such an operation it is best to combine a team of surgeons encompassing of a craniofacial surgeon, neurosurgeon and ophthalmologist. By making a coronal incision in the hairy part of the temporal and the frontal region bilaterally, the frontal bone is bilaterally deperiosted, including the superior and the lateral orbital margin (Figure 14 A, B). During this procedure the supraorbital and the supratrochlear nerves and blood vessels must be preserved. This is followed by osteotomy of the part of the frontal bone performed bilaterally, by using neurosurgical technique, and this part of the bone has been temporary removed (Figure 14 B, C).

Through this opening the base of the brain is lifted off the skull base and the orbital roof (Figure 14D). By a suitable raspatory, the superior, medial and lateral orbital walls are freed from the periosteum and orbital contents deep down to the level of fusion of the posterior and the middle third of the orbit (Figure 14E). The infraorbital margin is reached by the subciliary incision on the lower eyelid, the infraorbital part of the maxilla and the zygomatic bone is deperiosted, as well as the orbital floor deep down to the level of fusion of the posterior and the middle third of the orbit (Figure 14F). In the course of this operation it is necessary to perform bilateral desinsertion of the medial and the lateral ligament and to lift the lacrimal sac from its place, while preserving the continuity with the nasolacrimal duct. During the same procedure the nasal crest must be deperiosted. The infraorbital neurovascular bundle must be isolated and preserved. This is followed by orbital osteotomy performed by the intracranial and the orbital approach by using a small electrical saw or an adequate borer (Figure 14G, H). After the osteotomy of both orbits, the intact strip of the frontal bone, about 12 mm wide, remains supraorbitally between the two orbits and the opening on the frontal bone which is made at the beginning of the surgery (Figure 14G). This part of the bone is used for fixing both orbits in the new position. Upon performing complete osteotomy of both orbits, with removing the excess of the bone in the medial line and the nasal crest, and the excess of the bone on both sides of cribriform plate, mobilization of the orbits and their repositioning has been initiated. When the orbits are brought into a good position, they are fixed onto the supraorbital band of the frontal bone and also mutually by wire ligatures or mini micro plates (Figure 14I). For the purpose of improving ossification and preventing relapse, the bone fragments taken from the external table of the calvaria or the hip bone are placed into the empty space between the orbits and the adjacent bone. The frontal bone is returned to its position and fixed to the adjacent bone. Medial canthopexy is performed by interconnecting both medial ligaments through a bilateral fenestration on the nasal root. The lateral ligaments are fixed to the lateral orbital margin. Then the scalp is returned to its position and stitched in the usual manner. The method described has several modifications.

In cases of orbital dystopia various surgical procedures may be applied – depending on the type of dystopia. If the orbit is positioned laterally it is moved medially by a unilateral surgical procedure performed in cases of hypertelorism. In a similar manner, the orbit can be lifted, lowered or moved frontward. When the orbit is to be lifted, the part of the frontal bone which has been removed in order to lift the orbit shall be placed under the orbit in order to fill the empty space. The opposite procedure is used when it is necessary to lower the orbit.

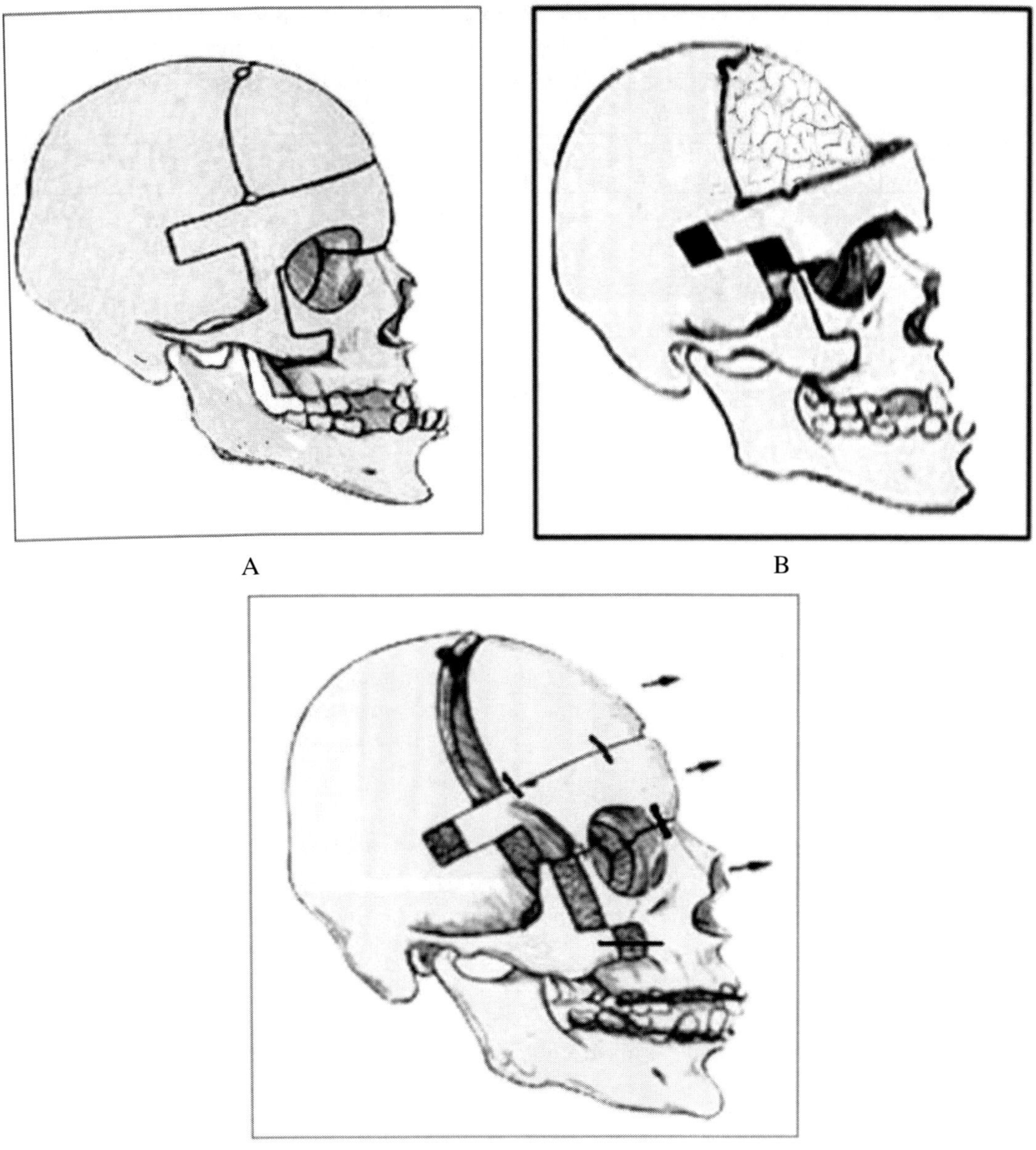

A B

C

Figure 15. A. Osteotomic incisions of the upper and the middle third of the face and the orbit for the purpose of correcting malformations in these regions, i.e., pulling the facial skeleton frontwards. These incisions are performed by using the coronal, the subciliary and the oral approach. B. The supraorbital part of the frontal bone has been pulled out bilaterally into a new, normal position and it serves as the point of orientation for the position of the upper and the middle third of the face C. The skeleton of the middle third of the face and the frontal bone are moved frontwards and fixed to the adjacent bones and also mutually fixed by mini i.e., micro plates. In the defects between the facial bones moved frontwards and the surrounding bones, for the purpose of improving ossification and preventing relaps, bone grafts are placed which are taken from the hip or calvaria.

In cases of craniofacial synostosis with skull deformities, hypoplasia of the middle third of the face and a marked eye protrusion (due to shallow and short orbits), the correction of facial, cranial, orbital anomalies and the eye protrusion requires performance of osteotomy of the frontal bone, both orbits and the skeleton of the middle third of the face. All the bones must be brought into a normal position (Figure 15). The method displayed in Figure 15 has several modifications which are applied depending on the specific case. Together with osteotomic cuts shown in Figure 15, nowadays special orthopaedic devices have been successfully used for pulling out, distraction of the bones after performed osteotomy. This is similar to a distraction of long bones by using the Ilizarov method.

6.6. Patients and Surgical Treatment Results

Craniofacial malformations in Serbia are relatively rare. Even in cases where it is possible to achieve good results by introducing surgical therapy, parents are often advised not to accept this type of therapy. Due to all these reasons, there was no opportunity for performing large number of operations in the field of craniofacial anomalies associated with the orbital anomalies.

In three patients who had “big eyes”due to slightly shallower and shorter orbits, excellent results were achieved by the surgical enlargement of the orbital volume (Figures 1, 2).

In six patients with microorbitism, due to anophthalmia that occurred after an early enucleation of the bulbus, by correction of the eyelids, the conjunctival sac and the orbital walls, conditions for the application of eyelid prosthesis are created.

In one patient with the clefts No.3 and No.4 according to Tessier, the reconstruction of the facial tissues and of the half of the nose was performed, as well as the correction of major coloboma of both eyelids, and also the reconstruction of the medial orbital wall and the orbital floor with lifting the eye by 8 mm and the correction of telecanthus (Figure 7). In five patients with Treacher Collins’ syndrome (clefts 6, 7, 8 according to Tessier), excellent results were achieved after performing complicated and complex craniofacial operations with the correction of anomalies on the orbit (Figures 8, 9).

Four out of twelve patients with Romberg’s disease had a marked enophthalmos in addition to the infraorbital region atrophy. Correction of the enophthalmos and the infraorbital region by using the rib cartilage or calvarial bone and the vascularized pericranial, galeoperiostal flap gave good results (Figures 10, 11).

The parents of a patient with trigonocephaly and hypotelorism due to a synostosis of the frontal, metopic suture refused the surgical procedure.

In two patients with plagiocephaly caused by unilateral synostosis of the coronary suture, the surgical procedure gave excellent results (Figure 12). A child with a monstrous anomaly – a marked Crouzon syndrome and hypertelorism – died a month after an extensive and complicated operation. The cause of death was meningitis. A young man with Apert syndrome with marked protrusion of both eyes, after a detailed preparation, got scared and withdrew from the complicated operation- osteotomy of the bones of the upper and the middle third of the face, with bilateral orbital osteotomy and movement of all the bones frontward (Figure 13). However, these types of surgeries were performed on other patients with facial hypoplasia in whom there were no changes on the orbits.

Conclusion

Congenital malformations of the orbit are most often associated with various malformations of the craniofacial region, i.e., they often represent a part of another congenital syndrome of the craniofacial region. That is why the surgical correction of those malformations is very complicated and requires knowledge of ophthalmology, orbital surgery as well as of craniofacial surgery. Using medern contemporary metods of orbital and craniofacial surgery, in most cases, a good team of surgeons, consisting of a craniofacial surgeon, neurosurgeon and an ophthalmic surgeon, is capable to achieve satisfying results.

References

[1] Bite V., Jackson I. T., Forbes G. S., Gehring D. G., Orbital volume measurements in enophthalmos using three-dimensional CT imaging, *Plast Reconstr. Surg*. 75: 502 – 507, 1985.

[2] Cedars M. G., Toth B.A., Expansion of micro-orbit using tissue expanders, in: Toth B. A. Keating R. E., Stewart W. B., An atlas of orbitocranial surgery, Martin Dunitz, London, 1999.

[3] Heinz G. W., Cepela M. A., Nunery W.R., The effect of maturation on the ability to stimulate orbital growth using tissue expanders in the anophthalmic cat orbit, Ophthal. *Plast. Reconstr. Surg*. 13: 115 – 128, 1997.

[4] Jackson I. T., Murno I. R., Salyer K. E., Whitaker L. A., Atlas of craniomaxillofacial surgery, Mosby, St. Louis, 1982.

[5] Jovanović S., Keros P., Cvetković D., Jeličić N., Vinter I., Eye Cavity and the Organ of Vision, Scientific Book, Belgrade, 1989.

[6] Kawamoto H.K., Rare craniofacial cleft, in: McCarthy J.G., Plastic Surgery, Vol. 4, Saunders, Philadelphia, 1990.

[7] Kennedy R. E., The effect of early enucleation on the orbit in animals and humans, *Am. J. Ophthalmol*. 60: 277-306, 1965.

[8] Koorneef L., Sectional anatomy of the orbit, Aeolus Press, Amsterdam, 1981.

[9] Manson P. N., Raus E.J., Iliff N. T., Deep orbital reconstruction for correction of post-traumatic enophthalmos, *Clin. Plast. Surg*. 14: 113-121, 1987.

[10] Marchac D., Surgical enlargement of anophthalmic-socket, in: Toth B. A., Keating R. F., Stewart W. B., An atlas of orbitocranial surgery, Martin Dunitz, London, 1990.

[11] Marchac D., Renier D., Craniofacial Surgery for Craniosynostosis, Little, Brown, Boston, 1982.

[12] McCarthy J. G., Epstein F.J., Wood-Smith D., Craniosynostosis, In: McCarthy J. G., Plastic Surgery, Vol. 4, Saunders, Philadelphia, 1990.

[13] Montodon D., Maillard G.F., Morax S., Garey L. J., Plastic and Reconstructive Surgery of the Orbitopalpebral Region, Churchill Livingstone, Edinburgh, 1990.

[14] Osborne D., Harden O.B., Deeming L.W., Orbital growth after childhood enucleation, *Am. J. Ophthalmol*. 77: 756 -764, 1974.

[15] Rončević R., Rončević D., Mandibulofacial dysostosis: Surgical treatment, *J. Craniofac. Surg*. 7: 280 – 283, 1996.

[16] Rončević R., Rončević D., Surgical reduction of "Big Eyes," Aesth. *Plast. Surg*. 21: 339 -341, 1997.

[17] Rončević R., Rončević D., Extensive traumatic fractures of the orbit in war and peace time, *J. Craniofac. Surg*. 10: 284 -300, 1999.

[18] Rončević R., Stajčić Z., Hanhart's syndriome with facial asymmetry, *Br.J. Plast. Surg*. 48: 511-514, 1995.

[19] Rončević R., Stajčić Z., Correction of facial deformities with pericranial and osteopericranial flaps, *Br. J. Plast. Surg*. 47: 230-234, 1994.

[20] Tessier P., Osteotomies totales de la face. Syndrome de Crouzon. Syndrome d' Apert. Oxycéphalies. Scaphocéphalies. Turricéphalies, *Ann. Chir. Plast*. 14: 207 – 214, 1976.

[21] Tessier P., Anatomical classification of facial, cranio-facial and laterofacial clefts, *J. Maxillofac. Surg*. 4: 69 – 92, 1976.

About the Author

Radmilo Roncevic, MD, DMD, PhD
Plastic, Reconstructive and Craniofacial Surgeon
The Clinic for Plastic and Reconstructive Surgery
Belgrade, Serbia
E-mail:ronac@eunet.rs

Dr. Radmilo Roncevic is one of the leading pioneers in surgery of the orbital cavity. He continues to serve as a consultant in plastic, reconstructive, and craniofacial surgery, a Professor of plastic and reconstructive surgery, and a sought after guest professor in the United States of America, Germany and Russia.

Index

M

N

O

P

R

S

T